THE FAT COUNTER GUIDE

Ronald M. Deutsch

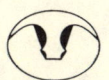

Bull Publishing Co.
P.O. Box 208
Palo Alto, California 94302

Trade Distribution by
Hawthorn Books, Inc.

Copyright 1978
Ronald M. Deutsch

ISBN-0-915950-16-2
Library of Congress
Catalog No. 77-21049

Contents

1 What the Fat Counter Can Do 1
2 Calories—Do We Need Fewer or More? 6
3 Protein—Do We Eat Too Much? 13
4 Carbohydrate or Fat—Which for Energy? 19
5 Vitamins and Minerals—Where the Balance Is 23
6 Making the Most of the Fat Counter 28
7 How to Use the Fat Counter 36
　Key Facts About This Table 43
　Tables 46
　Sample Diet Analysis 127

How This Book Came To Be
(A Special Acknowledgment)

In 1970, speaking to the first full meeting of the Society of Nutrition Education, I said that most of American's nutrition problems were due to misinformation that led to poor food choice. Fads and false ideas were causing people to seek just the foods of which they already ate too much, and to spurn just the foods they needed, in the mistaken belief that these were unhealthful.

As an example of a needed maligned food, I cited the potato. The nations' potato growers were interested. In 1973, The Potato Board launched a program dedicated to the kind of nutrition teaching I had been urging.

Through the years, the Potato Board has pursued its commitment—funding meetings and seminars, seeking better ways of nutrition education. From this work came a simplified system of food choice which I presented before the American Dietetic Association and the American Home Economics Association.

The concepts of these papers have become the book. The Potato Board has won many awards and kind words for its work in nutrition education. I want to add my applause for a contribution of a sort which is rare indeed in the commercial world.

R.M.D.
Laguna Beach
August, 1977

Introduction

This is the first simple guide to calorie counting which emphasizes fats. For years consumers have been told that proteins were good and carbohydrates were bad, and no one has said much about the part played by fats. Considering the facts, this is amazing.

A given quantity of fats contains more than twice the calories of the same amount of carbohydrates. Yet few people realize that most foods they think of as "high protein" are in reality high fat as well—and may supply far more calories than they realize. Since nutritionists generally agree that most Americans get ample protein and too much fat, it is indeed surprising that more attention has not been focused on the role of fats in the diet.

The facts are given simply, and beginning with the chapter, "How To Use The Fat Counter," the book provides an easy key to use of the tables which show where the fat calories are. The information will surprise many and provide keys to weight control and better health.

Helen Ullrich
Executive Director
Society for Nutrition Education

1
What the Fat Counter Can Do

The Fat Counter can help you reach almost any nutrition goal you choose—with the foods you like to eat. Do you want to:

- Control your weight?
- Include more fiber in your diet?
- Keep cholesterol low?
- Get the vitamins and minerals you lack—without costly pills or special foods?
- Cut down on saturated fats?
- Choose meals to meet the special needs of sports? Of pregnancy? The senior years? Childhood?

Whatever your nutrition aim, the Fat Counter can show you how to make the right food choices—from the restaurant menu, the supermarket shelf, or the party buffet. And because the final selection is yours, the food is always one you enjoy.

Moreover, there is a surprising health bonus. For when you use the Fat Counter, you automatically begin to reach other important nutrition goals.

How can the same simple guide to making food choices help us solve all of these problems at the same time?

On the surface, this might seem like a fanciful claim. But consider:

Virtually all of today's key nutrition goals can be met by following the same easy but flexible pattern of food selection. And for a simple reason.

Nutrition science boils down to two basic questions: What raw materials from food are required by our life processes? And which foods supply these needed substances in the right amounts?

We tend to follow a food pattern which supplies an excess of certain food chemicals and too little of others. For example, many of us choose foods which supply more bodily fuel (measured in calories) than we can burn. So we store the excess and grow fat. As another example, many of us choose foods with too little iron, and we become anemic.

The Fat Counter shows you a pattern of food choice which will help you meet your needs in a balanced way. It does this by showing what each common food supplies in the way of four basic nutritional factors—protein, fats, carbohydrates and calories.

Isn't that oversimplified? What about the vitamins, minerals, fiber and all the rest?

It is true that trying to balance precisely the needs of each individual against all of the nutrients in each specific food is an intricate matter.

For example, each of us needs some 50 different nutrients. And each of us needs somewhat different amounts—according to age, sex, height, weight, heredity, and scores of special circumstances from climate to lifestyle.

But luckily the human body can adapt to a considerable variation. And the characteristics of both people and foods tend to fall into a few fundamental patterns.

That is why nutritionists have been able to teach healthful eating with some very simple guidelines. For example, they use the Basic Four plan. This puts foods into just four groups—(1) dairy, (2) protein sources, (3) grains, and (4) fruits and vegetables. The concept works because certain clusters of essential nutrients tend to be found in each of these food groups.

But lately, the older food guides have begun to falter. For both our food supply and our styles of living and eating are changing dramatically. With a third of our meals being eaten away from home, and with much of our food for home consumption coming in pre-mixed, pre-fabricated forms, it becomes harder and harder to assign foods to the old nutritional groups. The Basic Four tends to stumble over a ready-made pizza or a frozen chicken pie.

Moreover, even when we can and do use the old nutritional groupings of foods, they often provide little help for some of our major problems. They do not, for example, deal with obesity.

The Fat Counter is designed to meet our most pressing nutrition concerns, in terms of the changes in the food supply and our newest styles of choosing food.

What pattern does the Fat Counter follow?

Despite many apparent differences in Americans' tastes and habits, and the bewildering variety of food products, there are some striking similarities in our diets. They are not all good.

Recent nutrition surveys have shown a certain strong pattern of error which seems to grow more clearly defined every day. It is a pattern of mistaken belief and misguided choice. And the key to a proper understanding is closely linked to the four nutritional factors—protein, fats, carbohydrates and calories—which are shown in the Fat Counter tables.

In the following pages, you will see how much of our nutrition trouble in America could be cleared up by a better understanding of how these four basic factors relate to our food and health. And you will see how to apply these factors to your own personal needs and problems.

By making good choices of proteins, fats and carbohydrates, you tend automatically to get more of the vitamins and minerals missing from many diets—such as vitamins A and B-6, iron and other trace minerals.

Nutritionists have realized for years that our choices of protein, fats and carbohydrates were going wrong—and that we were paying a high price in nutrition for the errors.

Recently, after several years of study, the U.S. Senate's Select Committee on Nutrition and Human Needs issued a recommendation on diet to the American people. It urged a shift in basic food choice, centering on the four fundamental factors you will find in the Fat Counter. These were among the principles urged:

Americans should limit their protein; they already consume much more than enough.

They should reduce their consumption of fats.

They should eat more carbohydrate—what we will see are called the "complex" carbohydrates.

These three simple guidelines can go a long way toward resolving most of our big nutrition problems. The Fat

Counter shows you how to put them to work—in terms of your own individual life and needs.

The next five chapters outline the reasons behind these basic concepts. Chapter 7 provides a simple chart for measuring personal energy (calorie) needs, and also tells how the Fat Counter works.

2
Calories—Do We Need Fewer or More?

Strange as it may seem, many modern nutrition problems begin with the fact that we don't eat as much as we used to.

This may seem odd to say in a time when we are all accused of overeating—when 20 to 40 percent of us are medically obese, and the rest of us are having a little trouble getting into our old slacks. But it is true.

Back in 1900, a male clerk of typical size—five feet nine inches tall and 154 pounds—burned and ate some 4,000 calories of food a day. Today, the same man would need only some 2,700 calories.

So our food consumption has declined about a third.

Isn't that decline a good thing?

In one sense, of course it is. The reason we need less food is that we are less active. If we ate as much as our forefathers ate, obviously we would all be fat.

But in another sense, that decline has caused some real problems. For a car or a furnace, fuel supplies nothing much more than pure energy to do work. But a human's fuel is something more.

In addition to energy, our fuel must also carry with it all the raw materials we need for growth, for making our own replacement parts, and for producing the many thousands of chemicals which we use to think, see and function in every way.

When we cut back our fuel intake, we reduce our supply of raw materials greatly.

But don't we need less of those raw materials when we do less work?

This is true of a few nutrients, such as certain B vitamins which are involved in letting us use our fuel.

But actually, our needs for the vast majority of nutrients remain unchanged. Theoretically, even if we were to lie in bed all day, we would still need just as much of most vitamins and minerals.

Couldn't we solve this problem by getting more exercise?

Most of us could certainly use more exercise. And it is true that the extra energy we would burn with that exercise would allow us to consume a somewhat greater quantity of food.

But only somewhat. Neither weekend sports, a morning's jog or daily setting-up exercises burn as much energy as you might think. Quite a brisk two-mile walk, for instance, costs the typical man only about 100 calories.

The activity levels of most Americans are generally classifiable as "light to sedentary." This includes such activities as:

Typing, sewing, ironing, auto and truck driving, paintting, lab work, playing musical instruments, walking moderately on a level, tailoring, pressing, garage work, electrical work, washing clothes, shopping, golf, sailing or table tennis.

If you do heavy work every day, increase your calorie allowance by about 10 percent.

To measure how weekend sports or a morning jog increase your calorie burn, you should take into account the length of time you spend doing them.

If you want to make such a calculation, use the chart on page 9. It shows the calories burned during one minute by different activities.

How much you weigh has a strong influence on this calorie burn. So notice the sample weights used here—154 pounds for a man and 128 pounds for a woman. If you weigh much more or less, you should modify the number of calories burned. For each 11 pounds extra you weigh, add 7 percent more calories, and subtract 7 percent for each 11 pounds less.

But even if we don't need as much food, isn't it true that most of us continue to eat far more than we need?

No, this is an exaggeration. And testing it can show us some basic facts about eating and fatness.

The energy that we get from the food we eat is, of course, measured in calories. Calories are not nutrients, but merely measures, like an ounce or an inch.

The calories of energy that we take in never disappear. They are either burned up or stored by our bodies as fat.

MEASURING SOURCES OF ENERGY

Calories Spent Per Minute

Activity	By a Man (154 lbs. or 70 kg.)	By a Woman (128 lbs. or 58 kg.)
Driving an automobile	.47	.43
Washing dishes by hand	.59	.52
Typing quickly	.59	.52
Ironing clothes	.59	.52
Washing floors	.82	.72
Doing light laundry by hand	.94	.82
Playing musical instruments at moderate rate	1.1	.92
Horseback riding, slow	1.1	.91
Painting, light work	1.2	1.0
Playing piano, fast	1.8	1.5
Walking, normal rate	1.8	1.5
Carpentry, average activities	2.1	1.8
Bicycling, easy rate	2.3	2.0
Canoeing, moderate speed	2.6	2.2
Vacuuming	2.6	2.2
Dancing, to moderate music	2.9	2.4
Skating, moderately	3.5	2.9
Swimming, moderate speed	3.5	2.9
Walking briskly (4 mph)	3.5	2.9
Riding horseback, at a trot	4.5	3.7
Ping pong, brisk game	4.6	3.8
Walking upstairs, moderate rate	5.3	4.4
Walking up 10% incline	5.3	4.4
Tennis, average rate	5.6	4.7
Heavy carpentry	6.0	5.0
Running, moderate speed	7.6	6.3
Bicycling, racing speed	8.3	6.9
Swimming hard (2 mph)	8.7	7.2
Dancing very vigorously	9.0	7.6
Running cross country	9.8	8.0

Adapted from various data, especially, Durmin and Passmore, FAO, and Foundations of Nutrition (Macmillan)

This is a basic survival mechanism of the body. For if we ran out of fuel for the brain, heart and other organs, life would stop. Just being late for dinner could be fatal.

So the body greedily stores every calorie of energy which we don't use.

Let's suppose that you eat a little extra every day, beyond the fuel you need—perhaps the equivalent of an ounce of prime steak. Calculating how this extra fuel is stored is easy. Some 3,500 calories equal a pound of body fat.

So if you ate that surplus ounce of steak—about 100 calories—you would add a pound (3,500 calories) every 35 days, or more than 10 pounds a year. In just a decade, you would weigh 100 pounds too much. From your twenties to your forties, you would gain some 200 pounds.

Clearly, very few of us average even 100 extra calories a day. The common excess girth of the middle years is more like 20 to 40 pounds.

Putting our mathematics in reverse, we can see that the overeating most of us do averages out to be very little extra indeed, perhaps 10 to 20 calories a day. Plainly, Americans are not gluttons. And it is equally plain that, to prevent obesity, we do not require radical changes in our diets.

(In actuality, few of us probably burn or eat so constant a number of calories. But the averages are still meaningful.)

If we can't eat the amount of food our ancestors did, how can we replace the nutrients we need?

There is just one realistic way. We must eat a more *compact diet*.

In a sense, the progress of modern life has led us to a very tight food budget—measured not in dollars, but in calories.

If we are to get adequate nutrition from our lesser food intake, we must learn how to spend our calories with care to get a good return of nutrients. Calorically speaking, we must look for nutrition "bargains."

Can't we ignore calories, and try to eat more foods of the kind that burn themselves up—or that don't turn into fat in our bodies?

If we could find such foods, nutritionists would probably be the first to rush and buy them. But, contrary to the widespread promotions and promises, there are no such foods.

For example, some people think that grapefruit contain enzymes which mysteriously burn up body fat. Alas, this is not true.

Others commonly believe that protein, unlike other energy sources in our food, is not converted to fat. This, too, is a completely false idea.

All nutrients which provide energy contribute to the total energy pool of the food we consume. If the total we take in is more than we use, so much more fat is formed.

The body is indifferent to the source of that energy—much as a fireplace does not care whether the heat of its fire comes from pine or oak.

However, it is true that, just as different woods supply different amounts of heat, so different nutrients supply varying amounts of energy. Protein and carbohydrate each furnish four calories from a gram. Fats provide nine calories for every gram.

Does this mean that, to get adequate nutrients from fewer calories, we have to get some of those nutrients from different foods than our ancestors depended on?

Exactly.

For example, in the 1870s, the average Englishman (and many Americans) ate perhaps a pound and a half of bread a day. This much bread could have supplied the whole quantity of protein needed by a man each day.

Similarly, the 1870s bread eater could have counted on his loaves for big contributions of some B vitamins, iron, and other nutrients. Bread could indeed be called the staff of life.

Today, many of us eat only a slice or two of daily bread. So even though much of our modern bread actually contains more of protein and of some vitamins and minerals, this source of food is no longer so important to us.

Theoretically, we could turn to bread for some of these nutrients, as our ancestors did. But in the necessary quantity, the price would be over 1,800 calories a day. No bargain here. So we must look to some other foods for the same nutrients.

Which foods can give us our needed calorie bargains?

The Fat Counter is designed to help you spot them, once you have a little more information.

Their number and variety is very large. The trouble has been that, in large part, our false ideas about the kinds of foods we need, and the quantities we need, have often led us to choose just the opposite.

As we look more closely at the facts about protein, we will begin to see how this problem arises.

3
Protein—Do We Eat Too Much?

Protein is certainly the most sought-after nutrient of our day, the darling of food ads and diet books. And all for no particularly good reason.

But isn't protein very important for health?

Immeasurably.

It is the stuff of life itself. Our heredity is spelled out in proteins. They are the very essence of our cells, of our blood and brain and muscle. They are the enzymes that control all the chemistry of our life processes. They are the hormones that trigger the actions of our glands and other organs.

Aren't these good reasons to look for more protein in our foods?

Not necessarily. Not if we are already consuming more than enough. And apparently, we are.

Recently, the Federal Trade Commission undertook a study to determine whether we needed any more protein. The FTC staffers concluded:

"Protein deficiency is evidently a rare nutritional problem in the U.S. . . . Every expert in the field of nutrition . . . expressed the opinion that 'the overwhelming majority of Americans get more protein than they require for good health from their usual diets.' "

Don't poorer people lack protein?

Not as a rule. If there were any vulnerability to lack of protein, we would expect to find it among the poor. For protein-rich foods—such as meats, fish, poultry—tend to be among our most expensive foods. The populations studied by the Federal government—in such projects as the massive Ten State Survey—dealt mostly with people at or near poverty income levels.

Yet even among our poor, protein consumption was found to approach *double* the amounts our bodies can use.

Won't extra protein, beyond our needs, make us healthier?

The Federal Trade Commission study was made to determine just this point—in order to judge the fairness of ads for protein supplements. Its poll of experts showed that there was no health value in extra protein. "The clear concensus of these experts," says the report, "is that protein supplements are a fraud on the American public."

Doesn't extra protein help to build muscle and improve sports performance?

Contrary to the belief of so many athletes and coaches, these ideas are untrue.

For one thing, activity scarcely increases our protein need, which is determined mainly by body size. Two people of the same size tend to have the same protein requirement, even if one gets far more exercise than the other.

In one typical study, cross-country skiers were checked to see how much protein they were using. They needed just as much while relaxing as they did during periods when they skied up to 50 miles.

Exercise is the only way to build muscle. As the muscle mass is increased, slightly more protein is needed. But that extra need is just a small fraction of the excess protein we all eat.

What happens to the protein which we don't need for building body structures and chemicals?

It is simply used, like fat and carbohydrate, as fuel. However, when protein is used as fuel, in a sense it does not burn cleanly. Waste products are left in the bloodstream.

Does high protein food have any special value for losing weight or preventing gain?

No, for as we have seen, the body merely treats the energy from protein as it does any other.

As a matter of fact, trying to control weight with protein may have an exactly opposite effect. For the problem is that there are very few true high-protein foods—mainly gelatine, blood, egg white, and some man-made protein extracts.

Then what are "high protein" foods really made of?

In most, the protein supplies only a fraction of the total calories of the food. And most often, the largest number of calories come from fat.

Consider a slice of prime rib roast—perhaps six ounces of cooked meat, separated from the bone. The calorie count for this slice is 748.

Of those calories, about 135 come from protein. Over 600 of the calories are from fat.

How fat rapidly builds up the calories of our meals can be seen by looking at the same slice of meat, with every vestige of visible fat trimmed away. There is still quite a little fat left. For much fat is concealed within the meat.

The trimmed slice now has only 410 calories, some 340 less. But more than half of those remaining calories still derive from fat and less than half from protein.

The point is not that one should avoid meat. It is that one problem with diets high in protein is that they tend also to be very high in fat.

Eggs are heavily used in many "high protein" reducing diets. And eggs, too, are excellent protein sources. A large poached egg, without added butter or margarine, has 82 calories. Of those only 26 are from protein; 52 are from fat.

Are vegetable source foods which are rich in protein lower in fats?

Some are, but the rule of thumb usually holds; where we find high concentrations of protein, we are likely to find goodly amounts of fat.

For example, nuts are among the richest vegetable sources of protein. A tablespoon of peanut butter has 94 calories, 16 from protein and 73 from fat.

Even soybean flours, unless some of the fat has been extracted, have more fat calories than protein.

Some beans and peas are high in protein but low in fat.

But here there are also ample amounts of carbohydrate, which dwarf the protein.*

Why do "high protein" reducing diets seem to work?

The failure to get enough carbohydrate changes our body chemistry to produce an illusion.

Trying to meet the body's energy requirements mainly from fat and protein produces waste products, especially those called *ketones*.

The great illusion of "high protein" diets begins as the kidneys try to flush these toxic wastes out of the body in urine. This takes a lot of water.

The loss of body fluid—which has nothing to do with body fat—can cause your body weight to fall some five to eight pounds within a matter of days. You are probably just as fat as ever, but drier. As soon as you return to a normal diet, the water returns, and you are plump and juicy again.

How much protein do we really need?

We will look at this in detail shortly. But for the moment, we might just note how well one of the foods we have just looked at meets our requirement.

---

*It should be noted here that not all protein is equally valuable in meeting body needs. Vegetable-source foods, such as grains and nuts, are lower in what nutritionists refer to as "protein quality" than are animal-source foods.

This is not to say that a vegetarian diet cannot be a good one. It is possible to get adequate protein quality from vegetable sources alone. However, eating some animal-source food is still the best shortcut to protein safety.

Not long ago, the Food and Drug Administration set a recommendation for daily protein to be used on food labels. That recommendation was far from minimal. It included large safety margins and was based on the needs of an adult male.

The six-ounce slice of prime rib roast, trimmed of fat, supplies 106 percent of his day's protein. Many other foods can do even better.

Clearly, adequate protein is not a problem for Americans.

4
Carbohydrate or Fat— Which for Energy?

Since Americans are among the world's biggest consumers of protein, it surprises many people to learn how small a part of our diet protein really is.

For despite the fact that we eat far more than we need—usually from two to four times Federal recommendations—protein provides only about 15 percent of our calories. Most of us could get along on about half as much.

Except for alcohol, this leaves only two important kinds of fuels to make up the bulk of our food—carbohydrates and fats. Together, they total some 85 percent of our diets, in terms of energy.*

So probably the biggest decision we make about our nutrition is the choice between these two fuels. That choice controls much of the nutritive quality of our diets.

Yet most of us are unclear about what carbohydrates and fats really are—and where they are found.

The Fat Counter shows us *where* they are.

---

*In terms of weight, water is the biggest ingredient of food—some 80 to 90 percent of the weight of most fruits and vegetables, 60 percent of meats and a third of even such "dry" foods as bread.

Aren't carbohydrate foods just so much sugar and starch—without much nutritive value?

Sugars and starches are the main carbohydrate fuels. Nutritionists frequently refer to grains, fruits, nuts and vegetables as "complex carbohydrate" foods. They distinguish them from simpler carbohydrate-rich foods such as table sugar, honey, and molasses. As we shall see, it is the complex carbohydrate foods which are generally short in our national diet.

There is a third main form of carbohydrate, which we usually can't digest—fiber. Fiber makes up most of the structural material of plants. It is seen as the strings in celery, for example, or the hull of grains, as in bran.

Together, these three groups—sugars, starches and fiber—are the main constituents of the whole world of plants. In other words, when we eat vegetables, fruits or grains, we eat mostly carbohydrates.

To believe, as some people do, that carbohydrates are harmful to eat, is to believe that mankind should not eat foods from plants. But those foods contain a lot more than just the sugar and starch which hold most of their fuel value.

For as we will see, all nutrients, even proteins, derive originally from plants. We may eat beef or drink milk. But the cattle from which we get the beef and milk initially took all their nutritional building blocks from the plants on which they grazed—that is, primarily carbohydrates.

To help us choose between fats and carbohydrates for fuel, has science set requirements for these two nutrients?

While some minimal requirements for health are shown, these are so small that no official *recommendations* are set by the Federal authorities.

In the final analysis, we must make our choices between carbohydrates and fat on another basis.

What about the illnesses which some people say carbohydrates can cause—such as "low blood sugar?"

Happily, these are largely figments of promoters' imaginations.

"Low blood sugar" is a symptom, not a disease. We feel it when we are hungry, since it is one of the signals by which our brain learns that we need to eat.

But "low blood sugar" is *not* known to be the cause of fears, nervous symptoms, sexual problems or psychoses.

Eating carbohydrate is *not* known to be the cause of heart disease or diabetes. True, diabetics have trouble with large amounts of sugar eaten in a short time. But since 1971, the American Diabetes Association has recommended a diet for diabetics which is higher in carbohydrate than in fat.

Carbohydrate is the basic fuel of life—not a problem for public health.

Should healthy people also eat more carbohydrate than fat?

All nutrition scientists are agreed that they should.

The most trusted authority on human nutritional requirements is the Food and Nutrition Board of the National Academy of Sciences. It sets the Recommended Dietary Allowances (the RDAs) which you see in nutrition textbooks.

In its most recent statement on human nutrition needs, the Food and Nutrition Board made this recommendation about the balance of our diets:

" . . . the proportion of energy derived from fat should not exceed 35 percent."

Since most of us get about 15 percent of our calories from protein,* this means that at least 50 percent of our calories should come from carbohydrate.

It is especially interesting that this is essentially the recommendation of the American Heart Association, and also of the Senate Report referred to in Chapter 1.

Let us see why.

---

*The Food and Nutrition Board's RDA for protein can usually be met by an adult diet which is no more than 8 percent protein.

5
Vitamins and Minerals—Where the Balance Is

One irony of the great current fascination with nutrition is that most of the vitamin and mineral worries of the public are not shared by scientists. And the concerns of science are not shared by the public.

For example: the public uses large amounts of extra vitamin E. But no vitamin E deficiency has yet been seen in the U.S. And excess vitamin E accomplishes nothing; it does not prevent heart and circulatory disease or sex problems; but it can cause some, if the excess is large enough.

Large amounts of vitamin C are far from harmless. And they do *not* prevent colds or flu. Moreover, scarcely anyone in the U.S. is seriously short of this vitamin.

Faddists and promoters even push "vitamins" which don't exist—such as B-15, B-17, vitamin "P" and vitamin "F."

Since vitamins and minerals can prevent or cure nothing except shortages of vitamins and minerals, what we do need to know is where they are really missing in our diets.

Which vitamins and minerals do Americans really lack?

In recent Federal studies, more than a third of children and many adults were short of vitamin A. Riboflavin (B-2) was often lacking, to a smaller extent. Many seem to be short of vitamin B-6, especially women who are on The Pill. And pregnant women and other groups tend to lack folic acid.

Iron is short among women, painfully short among many. A third of youngsters under age six are deficient enough in iron to show signs of anemia. And it appears that a number of trace elements—such as copper and chromium—may be too low in many diets.

Why have these shortages developed?

Many reasons are suggested. The decline in the amount of food we eat is one of the most important.

But along with this, especially in recent years, we have changed the balance of our diets by our choices of food. Our newer choices reduce our intake of certain vitamins and minerals, and also fiber. And they produce an excess of fat consumption that may be harmful.

What foods are we leaving out, to cause the shortages?

The most notable dietary change has been a shift in the way we choose between carbohydrates and fats—and how we choose foods within these two groups.

Since 1909, the Food and Nutrition Board finds that that part of our food energy which comes from fat has grown considerably—from 32 percent of our total calories to 42 percent. (For members of some socio-economic groups, the shift has been much greater.)

Meanwhile, our use of "complex carbohydrate" foods—such as vegetables, grains and fruits—has declined steadily, from 43 to 29 percent.

Isn't sugar taking up a lot of the space in our diets?

We do eat quite a little of the pure sugars, and as the Senate Report concluded, we must limit our sugar intake. (Otherwise, of course, we will use up too much of our calorie budget, leaving no room for complex carbohydrates, with their urgently needed vitamins and minerals.)

But for most Americans, by far the biggest source of excess calories is fat. Fat has replaced a lot of our valuable foods from plants. And a little fat can shove aside a lot of plant food.

A mere teaspoon of fat, for example, has the calories to replace a whole cup of broccoli. Often that fat carries no other nutrients with it. It may be in the oil of a bit more salad dressing, in one cookie—or a decision to fry a particular food.

The cup of broccoli (40 calories, mainly of sugars and starch) can provide almost 80 percent of a day's vitamin A, a fifth of the day's riboflavin, a modest amount of iron and some other trace elements.

Since the broccoli uses only two percent or less of the day's calorie budget, it is a nutritional bargain.

If we look at the "typical" woman's diet, we see that in the last 60 years or so she has lost some 300 calories of complex carbohydrate foods (as distinguished from pure sugar) from her daily diet. They have largely been replaced by fats—some 2.5 tablespoons.

For the calories in that extra fat she could have a quarter of a loaf of bread, a whole pound of potatoes, or seven or eight servings of leafy green vegetables.

Aren't the nutrients from plant foods also found in some fatty foods?

Some are, but some are not.

And even if we can get our vitamins and minerals from fatty foods, we pay a higher caloric price. To get certain nutrients—such as protein—from typical American foods, we *must* pay that price in fat calories. And we can afford to do so, provided we don't add still more fats unnecessarily.

Plant foods let us get more to eat with fewer calories. And we get not only a greater concentration of nutrients with each calorie, but we also get kinds of nutrients which are missing from our present diets. This is why using the Fat Counter can help us to close some of our vitamin-mineral gaps.

So the main reason to lower fat and increase carbohydrate is to get more vitamins and minerals?

Partly. But there is more.

Recently, we have heard much talk about the loss of fiber from our diets. That fiber comes from plants. Using more fat instead of complex carbohydrate food means closing out some of our fiber sources.

We have also heard that high intakes of fat, especially *saturated* fat, may contribute to heart and blood-vessel disease. A shift to carbohydrates automatically reduces intake of these fats.

We also lower our cholesterol intake. For cholesterol is not found in foods from plants.

How much do we need to reduce fats to accomplish this?

Less than you might think.

The American Heart Association recommends a ceiling of 35 percent of daily calories. For the average person, who gets some 42 percent of calories in fat now, this means a reduction of only about one sixth of current fat intake. Basic habits needn't change; and it leaves plenty of room in the diet for favorite fat-rich foods.

While it is still not entirely clear that eating more fats causes heart disease, or that eating less will prevent it, the Food and Nutrition Board agrees with the Heart Association about fat limits. For it sees the limits as a way to help solve many of our nutrition problems.

The Fat Counter can guide us to lower fat consumption without sacrificing a pleasurable diet.

6
Making the Most of the Fat Counter

When you put the Fat Counter ideas and tables to work you automatically make the principal changes nutritionists urge you to make.

When you transfer calories from fats to complex carbohydrates, you eat more from the two basic food groups neglected by most of us—vegetables and fruits, and breads and cereal grains.

Emphasis on these foods increases consumption of most of the vitamins and minerals generally lacking in our diets, such as hard-to-get B vitamins and scarce trace minerals. And of course, plant foods are our only sources of fiber.

In reducing fats, we tend to reduce saturated fats and cholesterol as well, thus responding to American Heart Association recommendations.

By seeing where the protein really is, and how little we really need, most of us can trim back a bit—at the same time trimming fats and our budgets. And we can add more variety to our meals. Just trimming the *size* of our meat portions can open up our plates to accommodate the corn, bread, potatoes, rice, peas, beans and noodles on which some of us have skimped needlessly—with no increase in total calorie cost.

Before you try to use the Fat Counter to improve your diet, however, you should know a few refinements of the system. Here are some of the most commonly asked questions about the Fat Counter—and some ways it can be employed by people with special nutrition needs:

Why does the Fat Counter show protein as "Percent of the U.S. RDA?"

To show you what the rich sources of protein are, and how easily you get far more protein than you can use.

U.S. RDA stands for U.S. Recommended Daily Allowance. (U.S. RDAs are derived from the Recommended Dietary Allowances, or just RDAs, discussed earlier.) The U.S. RDAs *are not* minimal amounts. They provide wide safety margins. The U.S. RDA for protein is derived from the desirable amount of protein for a typical adult male.

The Fat Counter lists protein content as "Percentages of U.S. RDA," so you can see how little protein-rich food it takes to get all the protein your body can use.

What if I am larger than most people?

You may need just a little more protein. However, if you are larger, you probably consume more total calories. So your consumption of protein is likely to go up, too. Check your diet to see what percent of the U.S. RDA you are getting now. It's probably more than double your need.

How far should I go with fat-cutting?

Keep in mind that the object is not to eliminate fats, but to trim them down where it's convenient to do so. We might say that the aim is *to make our fats count*.

To do this, we need only enjoy our fats, where we can, when they are accompanied by other important nutritive values. Our slice of beef is a good example. Trimming away all the visible fat carefully, we remove over 300 calories of fat, yet still get to savor the beef. And we get the important vitamins and minerals it contains, with the protein.

On the other hand, in some foods such as pork sausage, the fat is combined with the lean. Three one-ounce links actually have more calories than the trimmed beef. But while the beef supplies all our protein for the day, the three links of sausage provide only some 20 percent.

The classic example of getting the essential nutrition without the fat is in the difference between a cup of whole and skim milk. The whole milk has 159 calories. With the fats removed, the skim has only 88 calories. Yet the rest of the nutritive values of the milk remain.

Once we become aware of these simple fat-cutting devices, we find that goodly amounts of fat can be consumed for pleasure. A 170-pound man who limits his fats to 35 percent of his total calories can still have 1,040 calories of fat.

So I can still enjoy fatty foods?

Check the tables and you'll see plenty of room for pies and ice cream, for potato chips or nuts with a cocktail, or whipped cream on the pudding.

If we know where the fats are and make use of them in a knowing way, no food, no matter how rich, has to be sacrificed.

As an example, many calorie-conscious people feel they must skimp on butter. Suppose you have a choice between biscuits and toast. A one-ounce biscuit comes in at 103 calories. A slice of bread, weighing almost as much, offers only 63 calories. The nutrient values, otherwise, are similar.

The difference is 40 calories of fat. If that fat goes *into* the biscuit, we still want something on it. If we choose the bread we can use those calories for a pat of butter.

The secret of getting good nutrition from food without losing pleasure is control. Not self-control, which often becomes sacrifice in vain, when we don't understand foods and our needs. But the control of informed choice.

Aren't some carbohydrate foods much more nutritious than others?

Yes, they are. For example, green leafy vegetables are probably the biggest of all calorie bargains in terms of the nutrients they offer.

But in general, the rule should be to try and get a wide variety of carbohydrate foods—for each group has some special benefits.

Among carbohydrate foods, the starchy items have been the most neglected of late. For example, a potato can give you a large part of your needed vitamin C. It also includes useful amounts of iron, copper, vitamin B-6 and a number of other vitamins and minerals.

A reduction in "starchy foods" has been one of the most costly mistakes Americans have made in the last two decades, nutritionally speaking. They have developed an undeserved reputation for being low in nutrients. But in truth, some 85 percent of the world's people depend on these foods, not only for important segments of their vitamins and minerals, but for protein as well.

As the Food and Nutrition Board points out in its recommendations: "When intake of fat is reduced, it would be wise to substitute foods containing complex carbohydrates."

Should sweeteners be cut out of the diet to make it more compact?

Sweeteners are entirely acceptable foods, but they supply little except energy. It does not matter whether we speak of table sugar, brown sugar, raw sugar, honey, or maple syrup. Contrary to what can only be called superstition, none of these have any nutritive importance beyond their calories.

Like fat, these contributors of calories are luxuries when consumed with few other nutrients. And as with fats, we should cut those sources of sugar first which give us least nutrient return. If a child will eat a strawberry with a sprinkle of sugar, but won't eat this low-calorie source of some useful nutrients without it, chances are the sugar pulls its own weight.

Yet typical total American sugar consumption is over 400 calories per day. And over-all sugar consumption must be moderate, or else there won't be room in the carbohydrate calorie allotment for the foods which do provide other nutrients.

Do other nutrition guides, such as the Basic Four, still work when I use the Fat Counter?

They work together well. In fact, checking your food choices with the Basic Four groups, and with some modifications, is a good way to guard against missing important nutrients.

The Basic Four plan is this:

Milk Group

Two or more glasses of milk, servings of cheese, etc. daily. (Ice cream is in the milk group. But because of its fat and sugar content, it takes some 2.5 servings to equal the nutrient values of a glass of milk or a slice of cheese.)

Meat Group

Two or more servings a day of meats, fish, poultry, eggs—with dry beans, peas or nuts as alternates. (Note: In the last generation, there has been a decline in these alternates, due to the irrational concern about carbohydrates.)

Breads and Cereals

Four or more servings daily—either enriched or whole-grain. (Note: In the last generation, there has been some 17 percent decline in the use of wheat.)

Vegetables and Fruits

Four or more servings daily of vegetables and fruits— from a group comprised of dark green or yellow vegetables, citrus, tomatoes, potatoes, etc. (Note: Few Americans meet these recommendations.)

What can the Fat Counter do for the weight reducer?

It can let him custom-make his own diet—the most comfortable diet that will really work. Here's how:

- Set your calorie total below your daily need. (See p. 41) Don't be overambitious, however. It's hard to get adequate nutrition from diets under 1,200 to 1,500 calories. And you're not likely to stay on a diet on which you get too hungry. So it's best to start with about 500 calories a day less than you burn. In a week, you'll lose 3,500 calories—a pound.

- Check your diet for high-fat foods which are relatively easy for you to eliminate or cut down on. Look for protein sources which are lower in fat calories—for example, substitute fish or poultry for high-fat meats.
- Remember, you can cut 500 calories a day from your diet by eliminating less than two ounces of fat.
- Remember that complex carbohydrate foods (fruits, vegetables, breads and grains) have more water and fiber. They are *bulkier*. They allow you to eat a much greater *volume* of food with fewer calories, and more satisfaction.

How can the Fat Counter help in later years?

Since the senior citizen is likely to have a caloric need some 10 percent lower than that of the younger adult, this means that he must get his nutrients from a diet 10 percent lower in calories.

Trimming fats to the recommended 35-percent-of-calories-level will generally provide the necessary margin of safety.

How does the Fat Counter help in pregnancy and nursing?

The old wheeze that the pregnant or nursing woman can "eat for two" is badly misleading. She needs all the nutrients for both, but she does not need that many extra calories.

The Food and Nutrition Board estimates that, while pregnant, most women can use some 300 extra calories a day, an increase of some 12 to 15 percent. But pregnancy calls for a much greater increase in some nutrients.

Some of these increases offer no problem. For example, protein needs go up some two-thirds over normal requirements. But the 130-pound woman who already gets 15 percent of her calories in protein is already consuming the full amount she needs for pregnancy.

On the other hand, the pregnant woman's small increase in calories must include a third more of such nutrients as thiamin and zinc, half again as much of calcium and magnesium, and double the normal requirements for folic acid.

So she is faced with a need for a more nutritionally compact diet. She can afford still fewer of the dietary diluters, pure fats and sugars, than can the rest of us. Much the same is true of the nursing woman.

7
How to Use the Fat Counter

Using the Fat Counter is simplicity itself—mainly because the correction of our nutrition errors is so simple. For most Americans, that correction has two basic aims, which you should keep in mind as you use the Fat Counter. They are:

- To get a compact diet—one in which the calories are made to count to give you more nutrients.
- To shift the diet toward more of the foods that provide these nutrients which many of us are lacking.

To accomplish these aims, you must first establish some personal standards for your own diet. The first of these is the number of calories you want to eat each day.

How many calories do you burn?

The following table will give you a guide to how many calories it takes to maintain your present weight:

Your Weight (pounds)	Calories
Men	
120	2100
130	2275
140	2450
150	2625
160	2800
170	2975
180	3150
190	3325
200	3500
Women	
100	1560
110	1716
120	1872
130	2028
140	2184
150	2340
160	2496
170	2652

However, to personalize your calorie budget still more, you may want to take several factors into account.

1. *Your personal body chemistry* Some people's bodily machines use fuel more efficiently than others. So the average calorie number shown for your weight may be high or low. Only the scale will tell you whether your body uses more or less fuel than most people of the same weight. The averages used here are broad guidelines.

2. *Your age* Calorie needs decline with age, due to a

slowing of basal metabolism and to reduced activity. If you are over 51, reduce the calories by 10 percent.

3. *Your special activities*   The calorie expenditures used here are based on "light" activity. If you want to take into account the effects of daily or weekend exercise, see the chart on page 9, in Chapter Two.

4. *Pregnancy or nursing*   In general, pregnancy allows a daily increase each day of 500 calories.

5. *Childhood and adolescence*   These tables are all for adults only. The growth and greater activity of childhood and adolescence make demands for calories and nutrients which are not shown here.

Your calorie total becomes your daily "budget." The total calories shown for each food serving in the Fat Counter Tables show you how that food fits into that budget.

Measuring Maximum Food Fat

Since fat in foods is our main calorie extravagance, a second listing in the Fat Counter Tables shows you how many calories of fat each food serving contains.

Remember, nutritionists say that we should eat *no more than 35 percent* of our calories in fat. Once you know what your calorie total should be, you can take 35 percent of that number as your "fat limit." Or you can use the following shortcut table:

Total Calorie Budget	Fat Calorie Maximum (35%)
Men	
2100	735
2275	796
2450	856
2625	919
2800	980
2975	1041
3150	1103
3325	1164
3500	1225
Women	
1560	546
1716	600
1872	655
2028	710
2184	764
2340	819
2496	874
2652	928

Measuring Minimum Food Carbohydrate

Since nutritionists recommend that *no less than 50 percent* of our calories ought to be in carbohydrate, another Fat Counter listing shows the calories of carbohydrate each food serving provides.

Keep two key factors in mind here. First, that 50 percent is a *minimum*, not a recommended amount. Second, our need is for more fruits, vegetables and grains, the so-called complex carbohydrate foods.

You can either compute the 50 percent minimum of carbohydrate your diet should contain, or use the following shortcut table:

Total Calorie Budget	Carbohydrate Calorie Minimum (50%)
Men	
2100	1050
2275	1137
2450	1225
2625	1313
2800	1400
2975	1486
3150	1575
3325	1663
3500	1750
Women	
1560	780
1716	858
1872	936
2028	1014
2184	1092
2340	1170
2496	1248
2652	1326

Checking Your Protein Need

In general, it is not necessary to set a personal protein standard. As we have seen, the U.S. RDA for protein is set so high that it covers almost everyone's needs. That was its purpose.

The Fat Counter Table shows what part of the daily protein recommendation each food serving supplies.

Moreover, if you are at all like the typical American in your eating habits, chances are that your protein intake far exceeds your needs. Almost any day's food which you've eaten, or which you plan to eat, is likely to exceed the 100 percent goal.

You will quickly see that there is no point in adding up protein calories, and that is why the Fat Counter leaves them out.

Testing Your Diet with the Fat Counter

How good is your diet? You can learn a great deal about how well you are eating just by checking the food you ate or plan to eat in a day against the Fat Counter Tables. Simply fill in the chart below:

	Total Calories	*Total Protein*	*Max. Fat*	*Min. Carbohydrates*
Your Personal Need	————	100% U.S. RDA	————	————
Your Day's Food	————	————	————	————

Now compare your needs with what you ate. The answers, for most people, become strikingly clear. By making your foods match your needs—putting to work the refinements and suggestions outlined earlier in this book, and looking at the examples shown in the Sample Diet Analysis at the end of the Fat Counter Tables, you should be able to make substantial improvements in your nutrition.

The Fat Counter will help make those improvements possible and practical without the sacrifice of two of the most important elements in nutrition—pleasure and satisfaction. For any system of nutrition fails unless it is fully livable for a lifetime.

Key Facts About This Table

All Numbers Are Rounded Off.

To simplify reading food labels, Federal rules require that all food values be rounded off in a special way. This does not make the information inaccurate, because these values are actually only averages anyway.

The Numbers May Not Quite Add Up.

Don't worry. This comes from rounding off. Suppose a food has 103 calories. Data shows it has 3.12% of U.S. RDA of protein, 37.3 calories of carbohydrate, and 56.4 calories of fat.

Rounding off will show the values as 4% U.S. RDA of protein, 40 calories of carbohydrate, and 60 calories of fat, and a total of 100 calories. The slight resulting error has little meaning.

How Rounding Off Works.

The rules say that any number under 10 (calories, percent of U.S. RDA of protein, etc.) is rounded off to the nearest 2. Anything under 2 must either be shown as 2 or zero. Therefore, in the Fat Counter, any value more than 1.0 and less than 3.0 is shown as 2. Any value more than 3.0 and less than 5.0 is shown as 4, etc.

Once the number is over 10, the value must be shown to the nearest 5. So 16 is shown as 15. 22 is shown as 20.

When the number is over 50, it must be shown to the nearest 10. So 124 calories is shown as 120. So is 116 calories.

Where the Numbers Come From.

The basis of the Fat Counter is information from the U.S. Department of Agriculture's Agricultural Research Service, especially its Handbook No. 8 and Handbook No. 456. This is supplemented by analyses from individual manufacturers and marketers.

About Brand Names.

Brand names are not used. One reason is that, especially in mixed or prepared foods, the composition changes from time to time.

Convenience Foods Are Averaged.

Of the more than 15,000 products in today's supermarket, many are mixed foods. In the Fat Counter, two kinds of estimates are made about these foods.

For example, there are many kinds of frozen TV dinners based on fried chicken. They differ somewhat in how much meat, gravy, etc. they hold, and they change from time to time. So after comparisons of all available data, either averages are used or values are used for a single product which is typical of the group.

A second estimate is made on protein *quality,* when mixed. In many mixed products (say, a frozen beef pie) the processor will give a total figure for protein, but not his recipe. Knowing that the protein comes partly from meat (high quality protein) and partly from vegetables (lower quality protein), an estimate has been made of average protein quality, in order to show, by Federal method, how the product meets your needs.

Tables

	Protein* (% of U.S. RDA)	Carbohydrate Calories	Fat Calories	Total Calories
Abalone, raw, 3-1/2 oz.	40%	15	4	100
Acerola juice, 1 cup.	2%	45	6	60
Albacore (white tuna), 3-1/2 oz.	40%	–	50	130
Albacore (white tuna), raw, 3-1/2 oz.	60%	–	70	180
Alcoholic beverages. (See beverages.)				
Almonds, dried, 10 nuts.	4%	8	50	60
Almonds, roasted in oil, 1/2 oz., about 11 nuts, shelled.	4%	5	70	90
Almonds, shelled, slivered, 1/2 cup.	15%	45	320	390
Anchovies, canned, about 5, 3/4 oz.	8%	–	20	35
Apple, raw, whole, about 1/3 lb.	–	80	8	90
Apple, dried rings, 1/2 cup.	2%	120	6	120
Apple brown betty dessert, 1 cup.	6%	260	70	330
Apple butter, 1 tbsp.	–	35	–	35
Apple juice, 6 oz. glass.	–	90	–	90

*Protein, in terms of per cent of U.S. RDA (see p. 29), is included only so the reader can make sure that he/she is getting enough in the daily diet.

	Protein* (% of U.S. RDA)	Carbohydrate Calories	Fat Calories	Total Calories
Apple pie. (See pies.)				
Apple sauce, canned, unsweetened, 1/2 cup.	—	50	2	60
Apple sauce, canned, sugar added, 1/2 cup.	—	120	2	130
Apricot, raw, 1, about 1/12 lb.	—	20	2	20
Apricots, canned, unsweetened, 3 halves and liquid.	2%	30	2	30
Apricots, canned, in heavy syrup, 3 halves and syrup.	2%	80	2	80
Apricots, 3 dried halves, medium size.	2%	30	2	30
Apricot nectar, 6 oz. glass.	2%	110	2	110
Artichoke, boiled, 1, 10 oz.	6%	50	2	60
Artichoke hearts, canned, 3-1/2 oz.	2%	20	2	25
Asparagus, fresh, frozen or canned, 1/2" diam., 4 spears.	2%	10	4	15
Asparagus, frozen cuts, cooked, 2/2 cup.	6%	15	2	30
Asparagus, frozen spears, in hollandaise sauce, 3-1/2 oz.	6%	15	80	100
Avocado, medium size, 1/2.	4%	15	130	140
Bacon, broiled or fried, sliced medium thick (20 slices per lb.), 2 slices.	8%	2	70	90

*See note, p. 46.

	Protein* (% of U.S. RDA)	Carbohydrate Calories	Fat Calories	Total Calories
Bacon, Canadian style (back), 2 slices, 3-3/8" diam., 3/16" thick.	25%	–	70	120
Baking coatings for meat (shake-in-bag type), typical mix, 1 packet, 2 oz.	10%	140	45	220
Bamboo shoots, raw, cut up, 1/2 cup.	4%	15	2	20
Banana, common, 3-3/4" long.	2%	110	2	110
Barley, uncooked, 2 tsp.	6%	90	4	100
Basella (Indian spinach) raw, 3-1/2 oz.	4%	15	4	20
Bass, black, sea, meat only, 4 oz.	50%	–	10	110
Bass, small or large mouth, meat only, 4 oz.	50%	–	30	120
Bavarian Cream (orange, lemon, etc.), 1 cup.	8%	160	130	300
Beans, white, with pork and tomato sauce, canned, 2/3 cup.	15%	130	40	170
Beans, white, with pork and sweet sauce, canned, 2/3 cup.	15%	140	70	260
Beans, white, without pork, canned, 2/3 cup.	15%	160	8	210
Beans, red kidney, canned, 2/3 cup.	15%	110	6	170
Beans, lima, dried, cooked, 2/3 cup.	15%	90	6	130

*See note, p. 46.

	Protein* (% of U.S. RDA)	Carbohydrate Calories	Fat Calories	Total Calories
Beans, lima (Fordhook or thick-seeded), frozen, cooked, 2/3 cup.	10%	90	2	110
Beans, lima, frozen in butter sauce, 3-1/2 oz.	8%	70	25	120
Beans, mung, sprouted seeds, uncooked (bean sprouts), 1/2 cup.	4%	30	2	45
Beans, green snap, fresh or canned, cooked, 2/3 cup.	2%	20	2	20
Beans, green snap, frozen, cooked, 2/3 cup.	2%	20	–	25
Beans, yellow or waxed, canned, 2/3 cup.	2%	20	2	20
Beans, green, with almonds, frozen, 2/3 cup.	6%	35	35	70
Beans and frankfurters, canned, 1 cup.	15%	130	160	370
Bean soup, with bacon, canned, 1/3 can serving.	10%	70	40	150
Bean soup, with meat, homemade, 1 cup.	10%	100	130	260
Beechnuts, shelled, 1 oz.	8%	25	130	160
Beef, chuck, cut up for stew, with fat, cooked, 1 cup.	80%	–	300	460
Beef, chuck, cut up for stew, lean, fat trimmed, cooked, 1 cup.	90%	–	120	300
Beef, chuck rib roast or steak, boneless, choice, with fat, 4" × 2", 1" thick, 6 oz.	80%	–	560	730

*See note, p. 46.

	Protein* (% of U.S. RDA)	Carbohydrate Calories	Fat Calories	Total Calories
Beef, chuck rib roast or steak, boneless, choice, as above, but fat trimmed, 6 oz.	110%	–	200	420
Beef, chuck rib roast or steak, boneless, good grade, size as above, with fat, 6 oz.	90%	–	460	640
Beef, chuck rib roast or steak, boneless, good grade, size as above, fat trimmed, 6 oz.	110%	–	160	370
Beef, chuck roast or steak (arm and roundbone cuts), choice, with fat, 2 pieces, each about 2-1/2" square and 3/4" thick, 6 oz.	100%	–	290	490
Beef, chuck rib roast or steak (arm and round-bone cuts), 2 pieces as above, 6 oz., fat trimmed.	120%	–	110	330
Beef, chuck rib roast or steak, as above, good grade, with fat, 6 oz.	110%	–	220	430
Beef, chuck roast or steak, good grade, as above, but fat trimmed, 6 oz.	120%	–	80	300
Beef, flank steak (London broil), choice, 5" × 2-1/2" × 3/4", 6 oz.	120%	–	110	330

*See note, p. 46.

	Protein* (% of U.S. RDA)	Carbohydrate Calories	Fat Calories	Total Calories
Beef, frozen dinner, about 11 oz.	70%	120	100	320
Beef loin (porterhouse steak), choice, broiled, with fat, edible yield from untrimmed 1 lb. raw, 10.6 oz.	130%	–	1140	1400
Beef loin (porterhouse steak), as above, but fat trimmed, yield from untrimmed 1 lb., 6.1 oz.	120%	–	160	390
Beef loin (T-bone steak), choice, broiled, with fat, edible yield from 1 lb. raw, about 10.4 oz.	130%	–	1150	1400
Beef loin (T-bone steak), as above, but fat trimmed, edible yield from untrimmed 1 lb. raw, about 5.8 oz.	110%	–	150	370
Beef loin (club steak), choice, broiled, with fat, edible yield from 1 lb. raw, about 9.8 oz.	130%	–	1020	1260
Beef loin (club steak), as above, but fat trimmed, edible yield from untrimmed 1 lb. raw, about 5.7 oz.	110%	–	190	390
Beef loin, end or sirloin, wedge and roundbone sirloin steak, choice, broiled, 5″ × 2-3/4″ × 3/4″, with fat, 6 oz.	90%	–	490	660

*See note, p. 46.

	Protein* (% of U.S. RDA)	Carbohydrate Calories	Fat Calories	Total Calories
Beef loin, end or sirloin, wedge and roundbone sirloin steak, as above, fat trimmed, 6 oz.	120%	–	120	350
Beef loin, double-bone or flat-bone steak, choice, broiled, with fat, 2 pieces, each 2-1/2" square, 3/4" thick, 6 oz.	80%	–	530	700
Beef loin, double-bone or flat-bone steak, as above, fat trimmed, 6 oz.	120%	–	150	370
Beef, plate beef, simmered, with fat, edible yield from 1 lb. with bone, about 9.3 oz.	130%	–	890	1140
Beef, plate beef, as above, fat trimmed, edible yield from untrimmed 1 lb. with bone, 5.7 oz.	110%	–	110	320
Beef, rib roast, choice, roasted, with fat, 2 pieces, each 4" × 2" × 1/2" thick, total 6 oz.	80%	–	600	750
Beef, rib roast, as above, fat trimmed, 6 oz.	110%	–	210	410
Beef, round steak braised, broiled or sauteed, choice, with fat, 4" × 2" × 1" thick, 6 oz.	110%	–	240	440
Beef, round steak, as above, fat trimmed, 6 oz.	120%	–	90	320

*See note, p. 46.

	Protein* (% of U.S. RDA)	Carbohydrate Calories	Fat Calories	Total Calories
Beef, rump roast, choice, roasted, with fat, 2 pieces, each 4″ × 2″ × 1/2″ thick, 6 oz.	90%	–	420	590
Beef, rump roast, as above, but fat trimmed, 6 oz.	110%	–	140	350
Beef, ground, lean, 10% fat, fried to well-done, yield from 4 oz. patty raw, 3 oz. cooked.	50%	–	90	190
Beef, ground, as above, except medium lean, about 21% fat, 3 oz. cooked.	40%	–	150	240
Beef extender, "helper" or "one-skillet" meal mixes to which ground meat is added, about 1/5 of package. (Average values.)	8%	120	20	160
Beef, corned, boneless, cooked, yield from 1/2 lb. raw meat, about 5-1/2 oz.	80%	–	420	570
Beef, corned, canned, slice 3″ × 2″ × 3/4″ thick, 3 oz.	45%	–	90	170
Beef, creamed chipped, frozen entrée, prepared, about 5 oz.	30%	35	35	130
Beef stew, canned, 1 cup, about 7-1/2 oz.	30%	70	80	200
Beef stew, frozen, 16 oz.	75%	170	210	360

*See note, p. 46.

	Protein* (% of U.S. RDA)	Carbohydrate Calories	Fat Calories	Total Calories
Beef, sliced with gravy, frozen entrée, about 5 oz.	45%	15	60	160
Beef pot pie, frozen, 8 oz. individual pie.	25%	160	180	400
Beets, common red, fresh, boiled, peeled, 2 (2" diam.).	2%	30	–	30
Beets, canned, drained solids, 1/2 cup.	2%	30	–	30
Beets, harvard, canned, 1/2 cup.	2%	70	–	80
Beets, pickled, canned, 1/2 cup.	2%	70	–	80
Beet greens, cooked, 1 cup.	4%	20	2	25
Beverages, alcoholic				
Bourbon, gin, rum, vodka, blended whiskey, 1-1/2 oz. jigger, 86 proof.	–	–	–	110
Bourbon, gin, rum, vodka, blended whiskey, 1-1/2 oz. jigger, 100 proof. (Calories derive from alcohol).	–	–	–	120
Beer, 4.5% alcohol, 12 oz. can.	2%	55	–	150
Wine, table, about 12% alcohol (as Burgundies, Rhine wines, Cabernets, Pinots, Roses, Chiantis, etc.), typical wine glass serving, about 3-1/2 oz.	–	15	–	90

*See note, p. 46.

	Protein* (% of U.S. RDA)	Carbohydrate Calories	Fat Calories	Total Calories
Wine, fortified types, about 19% alcohol (as Sherry, Port, Madera, Marsala) as well as certain sweet dessert wines, wine glass serving, 3-1/2 oz.	–	32	–	140
Wine, fortified and dessert types, as above, sherry glass serving, 2 oz.	–	15	–	90
Biscuits, baking powder, home recipe, enriched or self-rising flour, 1 biscuit, 2" diam.	3%	50	45	100
Biscuits from mix, made with milk, 1 biscuit, 2" diam.	3%	60	25	90
Biscuits, frozen or chilled, heat and serve, most types, 1 biscuit.	2%	40	20	60
Blackberries, fresh, 1/2 cup.	1%	40	6	45
Blackberries, canned, water pack, unsweetened, 1/2 cup.	1%	45	6	50
Blackberries, canned 1/2 cup, in heavy syrup.	1%	110	6	120
Blackberries, frozen, unsweetened, 1/2 cup.	1%	30	2	30
Blackberries, frozen, sweetened, 1/2 cup.	1%	70	2	70
Blackberry juice, canned, unsweetened, 3/4 cup.	1%	60	10	70
Blackeye peas (cowpeas), fresh or canned, 1/2 cup.	12%	60	6	90

*See note, p. 46.

	Protein* (% of U.S. RDA)	Carbohydrate Calories	Fat Calories	Total Calories
Blackeye peas, frozen, cooked, 1/2 cup.	15%	80	4	110
Blueberries, fresh or frozen, unsweetened, 1/2 cup.	1%	45	4	45
Blueberries, frozen, sweetened, 1/2 cup.	1%	120	4	120
Bluefish, baked or broiled with butter or margarine, fillet, about 7-3/4" × 4" × 3/4" (5.5 oz.).	90%	–	70	250
Bluefish, breaded, fried, fillet, size as above.	78%	30	140	320
Blood sausage (blood pudding), or blood and tongue sausage, 1 oz. Approx. 3/8" thick slice from a round 2-1/4" diameter, or a half slice from loaf shape, 5" × 4" × 1/8".	9%	–	90	110
Bockwurst, 1 link, about 2.3 oz.	16%	2	140	170
Bologna, slice, about 4-1/2" diameter, 1/8" thick, made with binders, variety meats, etc.	8%	2	70	90
Bologna, slice as above, all meat, or with nonfat dry milk, 1 oz.	8%	4	60	80
Boston brown bread, canned, slice, 3-1/4" diameter, 1/2" thick.	4%	80	6	100
Bouillon cubes, about 1/2".	1%	1	1	5

*See note, p. 46.

	Protein* (% of U.S. RDA)	Carbohydrate Calories	Fat Calories	Total Calories
Boysenberries. (See values for blackberries, above.)				
Bran, cereal, added sugar, salt, malt extract, vitamins, 1/2 cup.**	5%	50	8	70
Bran flakes (40% bran), added sugar, 1 cup.	5%	90	6	110
Bran flakes with raisins, added sugar, 1 cup.	6%	120	6	140
Braunschweiger, 1 slice, about 2-1/2" diameter, 1/4" thick.	6%	2	45	60
Brazil nuts, 6 large or 8 medium, about 1 oz.	6%	10	170	190
Bread, cracked wheat, fresh or toasted, 1 slice, about 1 oz.	3%	50	6	70
Bread, French or Vienna, enriched or unenriched, 1 slice, about 1 oz. (Also, see **rolls.**)	4%	60	8	70
Bread, Italian, enriched or unenriched, 1 slice, about 1 oz.	4%	70	2	80
Bread, raisin, fresh or toasted, 1 slice, about 1 oz.	3%	50	6	70
Bread, rye, American style (2/3 wheat flour, 1/3 rye flour), 1 slice, about 1 oz.	4%	50	2	60

*See note, p. 46.

** Much of the carbohydrate of bran is indigestible. Carbohydrate calories shown are those estimated for the digestible portion.

	Protein* (% of U.S. RDA)	Carbohydrate Calories	Fat Calories	Total Calories
Bread, pumpernickel, 1 slice, 1 oz.	4%	70	4	80
Bread, salt-rising, enriched or unenriched, fresh or toasted, 1 slice, about 1 oz.	3%	50	6	60
Bread, sweet, from mix (as banana, date, etc.), typical piece, 2-1/2 oz. or 1/12 loaf.	4%	120	45	170
Bread, white, enriched or unenriched, fresh or toasted, 1 slice, about 1 oz.	4%	60	8	80
Bread, whole wheat, enriched or unenriched, fresh or toasted, 1 slice, about 1 oz.	4%	60	6	70
Bread pudding, with raisins, 1/2 cup.	12%	150	70	250
Bread sticks, 1 stick.	4%	30	2	40
Bread stuffing, from mix, prepared with water and butter or other fat, 1/2 cup.	7%	100	140	250
Breakfast drink when prepared with 8 oz. glass of milk, from commercial instant mix.	30%	150	80	290
Breakfast, frozen, sausage with pancake, waffle or French toast, about 6 oz.	35%	160	130	430

*See note, p. 46.

	Protein* (% of U.S. RDA)	Carbohydrate Calories	Fat Calories	Total Calories
Broccoli, fresh, cooked, 1 medium stalk.	9%	30	4	35
Broccoli, frozen, chopped, cooked, 1 cup.	6%	35	6	50
Broccoli, frozen, cooked, 3 whole spears, about 5" long, 3 oz.	4%	15	2	25
Broccoli, frozen in butter sauce, 3-1/2 oz.	4%	15	20	45
Broccoli, frozen with hollandaise sauce, 3-1/2 oz.	6%	15	80	110
Broccoli, frozen in cheese sauce, 3-1/2 oz.	8%	25	20	60
Brownies with nuts, (1-3/4" × 1-3/4" piece).	2%	40	60	100
Brussels sprouts, fresh, cooked, 1 cup, about 7 or 8 sprouts.	10%	40	6	60
Brussels sprouts, frozen, cooked, 1 cup.	8%	40	2	50
Butter, stick, 1/4 lb.	2%	2	830	830
Butter, 1 tbsp.	–	–	100	100
Butter, pat, 1" diam.	–	–	40	40
Butter, whipped, 1 tbsp.	–	–	70	70
Buttermilk, 1 cup.	20%	50	2	90
Cabbage, red or common, cooked or raw, 1 cup.	2%	25	2	30
Cabbage, spoon (or white mustard cabbage or pakchoy), 1 cup, leaves and stems, cooked.	4%	15	3	25

*See note, p. 46.

	Protein* (% of U.S. RDA)	Carbohydrate Calories	Fat Calories	Total Calories
CAKE: *2-1/2" arc of 2 layer, 9" cake unless specified otherwise.*				
Cake, angelfood, from tube pan, 1/12 of cake.	8%	150	1	160
Cake, Boston cream, 1/12 of 8" diam., 2 layer.	7%	140	60	210
Cake, chocolate devil's food, with chocolate icing.	7%	220	150	370
Cake, white or yellow, with icing.	6%	250	120	390
Cake, white or yellow, no icing.	5%	150	100	260
Cake, fruit, dark or light, 1 slice, 2" × 1-1/2" × 1/4".	1%	35	20	60
Cake, gingerbread, 1 piece, 3" × 3" × 2".	7%	240	110	370
Cake, pound, old-fashioned, 1 slice about 3-1/2" × 3" × 1/2".	3%	60	50	120
Cake, sponge, about 2-1/2" arc , 9" diam. tube pan.	8%	140	35	200
Cake-mix, angelfood, 2-1/2" arc. of a 9" tube pan.	5%	130	–	140
Cake-mix, coffee cake, made with eggs, milk, 1 piece, about 4" × 3" × 1".	10%	230	90	350
Cake-mix, devil's food chocolate, made with eggs.	6%	210	100	310
Cake-mix, gingerbread, 1 piece, about 2" × 2" × 1".	1%	50	15	70

*See note, p. 46.

	Protein* (% of U.S. RDA)	Carbohydrate Calories	Fat Calories	Total Calories
Cake-mix, white or yellow, made with eggs, not iced.	6%	240	90	330
CAKE ICING: *enough for 1/12 of 9" cake.*				
Cake icing, chocolate, home recipe.	1%	70	35	110
Cake icing, white, uncooked, home recipe.	–	90	15	100
Cake icing, white, boiled, home recipe.	–	70	–	70
Cake icing from mix, chocolate fudge.	1%	70	35	100
Candied cherries, 10, about 1-1/4 oz.	–	120	–	120
Candied ginger root, 1 oz.	–	100	–	100
Candied grapefruit, lemon, orange, citron, pineapple, 1 oz.	–	90	–	90
CANDY: *1 oz. servings.*				
Candy, butterscotch.	–	110	10	120
Candy corn (fondant), about 20 pieces.	–	100	5	105
Candy, caramels, plain or chocolate.	2%	90	25	110
Candy, caramels, plain or chocolate, with nuts.	2%	80	40	120
Candy, chocolate, bittersweet.	3%	50	100	140
Candy, chocolate, semisweet, about 10 small, cooking-size pieces.	2%	70	90	160

*See note, p. 46.

	Protein* (% of U.S. RDA)	Carbohydrate Calories	Fat Calories	Total Calories
Candy, milk chocolate.	3%	60	80	150
Candy, milk chocolate with almonds or peanuts.	6%	50	100	150
Candy, chocolate coated, coconut center.	1%	80	45	125
Candy, chocolate coated fondant, as in mints, etc.	1%	90	25	115
Candy, chocolate coated peanuts, 2 clusters or 8-16 single nuts.	7%	45	110	160
Candy, chocolate coated raisins, about 18-28 large raisins.	2%	80	45	120
Candy, fudge, chocolate or vanilla.	1%	90	30	120
Candy, fudge, chocolate or vanilla with nuts.	2%	80	45	120
Candy, gumdrops.	–	100	2	100
Candy, hard, as sour balls.	–	110	2	110
Candy, jellybeans, about 10.	–	110	–	100
Candy, marshmallows, about 4 regular size.	1%	90	–	90
Candy, peanut brittle.	2%	90	25	120
Cantaloup, 1/2, 5″ diameter.	3%	80	2	90
Carbonated beverages. (See type.)				
Carbonated water, unsweetened.	–	–	–	–
Carrot, raw, 1 carrot, 1″ diameter and 7″ long, about 5-1/2 per lb.	1%	30	–	30
Carrot, cooked, 1/2 cup of slices.	1%	20	–	25

*See note, p. 46.

	Protein* (% of U.S. RDA)	Carbohydrate Calories	Fat Calories	Total Calories
Carrot, dehydrated, 1 oz.	–	4	–	5
Carrots, frozen in butter sauce, 3-1/2 oz.	–	25	25	50
Carrots, frozen with brown sugar, 1/2 cup.	2%	70	20	90
Casaba melon, raw, wedge about 1/10 of melon, about 7-3/4" long, 2" wide at center.	3%	35	–	35
Cashew nuts, 1 oz., about 14 large kernels or 18 medium.	8%	35	120	160
Catsup, tomato, 1 tbsp., about 1/2 oz.	–	15	–	15
Cauliflower, raw or cooked, fresh or frozen, 1/2 cup.	2%	10	–	15
Cauliflower, frozen in butter sauce, 3-1/2 oz.	2%	10	25	40
Cauliflower, frozen in cheese sauce, 3-1/2 oz.	6%	25	25	60
Caviar, from sturgeon, granular, 1 oz., about 2 tbsp.	16%	4	40	70
Caviar, from sturgeon, pressed, 1 oz., about 2 tbsp.	20%	6	40	90
Celery, raw, large outer stalk, about 1-1/2 oz., about 8" long, 1-1/2" wide at the base.	1%	6	–	8
Celery, raw or cooked, chopped, 1 cup, over 4 oz.	2%	20	–	20

*See note, p. 46.

	Protein* (% of U.S. RDA)	Carbohydrate Calories	Fat Calories	Total Calories
Chard, Swiss, leaves and stalks, or leaves only, 1 cup, cooked.	4%	20	2	25
Charlotte Russe, made with ladyfingers and whipped cream, 1 serving, about 4 oz.	12%	150	150	330
Cheese, American type, 1 oz. slice.	15%	6	60	90
Cheese, blue or Roquefort type, 1 oz., about 1″ × 1″ × 1.6″.	14%	2	80	100
Cheese, brick, 1 oz., about 1″ × 1″ × 1.6″.	14%	2	80	100
Cheese, Camembert, wedge from 4 oz. package of 3 wedges, about 1-1/3 oz.	14%	2	90	110
Cheese, cheddar, 1 oz.	16%	2	80	110
Cheese, cheddar, shredded, 1 cup, 4 oz.	60%	10	330	450
Cheese, Colby, natural, 1 oz.	15%	4	80	110
Cheese, cottage, creamed (4.2% milk fat), small curd, 1/2 cup, about 4 oz.	30%	12	40	110
Cheese, cottage, 1/2 cup as above, but large curd.	34%	12	45	120
Cheese, cottage, **not** creamed, 1/2 cup.	30%	8	2	60
Cheese, cream, regular, small package, about 3 oz.	15%	8	290	320
Cheese, cream, regular, about 1″ cube, a little more than 1/2 oz.	3%	2	50	60

*See note, p. 46.

	Protein* (% of U.S. RDA)	Carbohydrate Calories	Fat Calories	Total Calories
Cheese, cream, whipped, half of prepackaged container, 2 oz.	10%	4	200	210
Cheese, Limburger, piece about 1″ × 1″ × 1.6″, about 1 oz.	13%	2	70	100
Cheese, mozzarella, 1 oz.	20%	6	40	80
Cheese, Parmesan, shredded, 1 tbsp., about 1/6 oz.	4%	–	12	20
Cheese, Parmesan, grated, 1/2 cup, not packed, about 1.8 oz.	47%	8	140	230
Cheese, Swiss, 1″ cube, a little more than 1/2 oz.	9%	2	40	60
Cheese, processed American, pasteurized, shredded, not packed, 1 cup, about 4 oz.	58%	8	310	420
Cheese, processed American, slice, about 3-1/2″ × 3-1/2″ × 1/8″ thick, about 1 oz.	15%	2	80	110
Cheese, processed Swiss, 1 oz. slice, about 3-1/2″ × 3-1/2″ × 1/8″ thick.	16%	2	70	100
Cherimoya, raw, 5″ diameter, 1/3 fruit, about 10 oz.	3%	160	6	160
Cherries, sweet, whole, 10 cherries.	1%	45	2	50
Cherries, sour, canned, solids and liquid, 1 cup.	3%	100	4	110
Cherries, sweet, packed in water, 1/2 cup.	2%	60	2	60

*See note, p. 46.

	Protein* (% of U.S. RDA)	Carbohydrate Calories	Fat Calories	Total Calories
Cherries, sweet, pitted and unpitted, packed in syrup, 1/2 cup.	2%	110	2	110
Chestnuts, fresh, shelled, 10 nuts.	3%	120	10	140
Chestnuts, shelled, 1 cup, about 6 oz.	7%	270	22	310
Chewing gum, 1 stick.	—	6	—	6
Chicken, light meat, without skin, 1 cup (about 5 oz.), chopped or diced, cooked.	100%	—	45	230
Chicken, dark meat, without skin, 1 cup, chopped or diced, cooked.	90%	—	80	250
Chicken, back, from fryer, about 2 oz.	27%	10	80	140
Chicken, half breast, from fryer, about 3.3 oz.	57%	4	45	160
Chicken, drumstick, about 2 oz.	27%	6	35	90
Chicken, thigh, about 3 oz.	33%	6	50	120
Chicken, wing, about 2 oz.	20%	4	40	80
Chicken, canned, meat only, 1/2 cup, about 3.6 oz.	50%	—	108	210
Chicken a la king, canned, 5.2 oz.	25%	35	110	190
Chicken a la king, home recipe, 1 cup.	60%	50	310	470
Chicken fricassee, home recipe, 1 cup.	80%	30	200	390
Chicken potpie, home recipe, 1/3 of pie, about 8 oz.	50%	170	280	550

*See note, p. 46.

	Protein* (% of U.S. RDA)	Carbohydrate Calories	Fat Calories	Total Calories
Chicken dinner, fried, frozen, 10-11 oz.	60%	190	110	410
Chicken livers in sauce, frozen entrée, 4 oz.	40%	15	35	120
Chicken and noodle frozen dinner, 11 oz.	35%	190	110	380
Chicken pie, frozen, 8 oz.	30%	100	220	430
Chickpeas (or garbanzos), 1/2 cup, dry.	40%	240	45	360
Chicory (endive, French or Belgian), 1 cup, chopped.	2%	12	–	15
Chili con carne with beans, canned, 1 cup.	35%	120	140	340
Chili con carne with beans, frozen, 8 oz.	25%	90	170	310
Chives, 1 teaspoon.	–	–	–	–
Chocolate, bitter or baking, 1 oz. or 1/8 cup.	4%	35	140	170
Chocolate candy. (See candy, chocolate.)				
Chocolate syrup or topping, thin type, 1 oz., about 2 tbsp.	2%	90	8	100
Chocolate syrup, fudge type, 1 oz., about 2 tbsp.	2%	80	45	130
Chop suey, meat, no noodles, homemade, 1 cup, a little more than 1/2 lb.	50%	50	150	300
Chop suey, frozen entrée, 7 oz. bag.	20%	40	40	120

*See note, p. 46.

	Protein* (% of U.S. RDA)	Carbohydrate Calories	Fat Calories	Total Calories
Chow mein, chicken, no noodles, homemade, 1 cup, a little more than 1/2 lb.	60%	40	90	260
Chow mein, chicken, no noodles, canned, 1 cup, a little more than 1/2 lb.	10%	70	2	90
Chow mein, shrimp, canned, no noodles, 1 cup.	15%	20	50	80
Cider. (See apple juice.)				
Clams, raw, meat only, soft, 1/4 pint, 4 oz., about 10 large, 13 medium, or 16 small.	35%	6	20	90
Clams, raw, meat only, hard or round, about 1/4 pint or 1/4 lb., chowder type, about 3; mediums, about 4-5; cherrystones, about 7; littlenecks, about 9.	30%	25	10	90
Clams, canned (type unspecified) 1/2 cup, drained solids only, about 3 oz.	30%	6	20	80
Clam liquor, broth, nectar, bouillon, etc., 1 cup, canned.	2%	20	2	45
Cocoa and chocolate-flavored beverage powder, with nonfat dry milk, about 4 heaping tsps. or 1 oz.	10%	80	8	100
Cocoa powder, no milk, as above.	2%	100	6	100

*See note, p. 46.

	Protein* (% of U.S. RDA)	Carbohydrate Calories	Fat Calories	Total Calories
Cocoa, dry powder, typical prepared, 1 tbsp.	2%	10	10	20
Coconut, fresh, grated meat, 1/4 cup.	–	8	60	70
Coconut milk (from meat and nut liquid), 1 cup.	12%	50	540	610
Coconut water (liquid from nut only), 1 cup.	2%	45	4	55
Cod, meat only, broiled with butter or margarine, 4 oz. (2 fillets, about 5″ × 2-1/2″ × 1″).	70%	–	50	190
Cod, canned, drained meat only, 1 cup, about 5 oz.	60%	–	4	120
Codfish cakes, fried, 1 regular size cake or 5 bite-size, about 2 oz.	20%	25	50	100
Codfish cakes, frozen, portion as above.	12%	40	100	160
Coffee, instant powder, regular and freeze-dried, 1 tsp.	–	2	–	2
Cola soft drinks, 8 oz.	–	100	–	100
Coleslaw, made with mayonnaise or homemade French dressing, 1/2 cup.	2%	25	140	170
Coleslaw, made with commercial French dressing or mayonnaise-type commercial salad dressing, 1/2 cup.	2%	18	40	60
Collards, fresh or frozen, cooked, 2/3 cup.	4%	20	6	30

*See note, p. 46.

	Protein* (% of U.S. RDA)	Carbohydrate Calories	Fat Calories	Total Calories
COOKIES: *diameter shown first and thickness second. Amount is for 1 cookie.*				
Cookies, chocolate-chip, about 45 per lb., 2-1/3".	–	25	30	50
Cookies, fig bars, square, about 1-5/8" × 1-5/8" × 1/2", about 32 per lb.	–	40	6	50
Cookies, gingersnaps, 2" × 1/4", about 64 per lb.	–	20	6	30
Cookies, ladyfingers, about 3" × 1-1/2" × 1" before split, about 41 per lb.	2%	30	8	40
Cookies, macaroons, 2-3/4" × 1/4", about 24 per lb.	2%	50	40	90
Cookies, marshmallow, chocolate coated, 1-3/4" × 3/4", about 36 per lb.	–	40	15	55
Cookies, oatmeal with raisins, 2-1/2" × 1/4", about 35 per lb.	2%	40	20	60
Cookies, sandwich type, creme filled, chocolate or vanilla, 2-1/4", about 45 per lb.	–	30	20	50
Cookies, sugar, soft type, 2-1/4", about 56 per lb.	–	20	12	35
Cookies, sugar wafers, 2-1/2" × 3/4" × 1/2", about 128 per lb.	–	10	6	20
Cookies, vanilla wafers, 1-3/8" × 1/4", about 150 per lb.	–	8	4	15

*See note, p. 46.

	Protein* (% of U.S. RDA)	Carbohydrate Calories	Fat Calories	Total Calories
Corn on the cob, fresh or frozen, boiled, 1 ear, about 5″ long and 1-3/4″ diam., white or yellow.	4%	65	8	70
Corn, kernels boiled, cut from the cob, fresh or frozen, 1/2 cup.	4%	60	8	70
Corn, canned, cream style, white or yellow, solids and liquid, 1/2 cup.	4%	100	6	110
Corn, canned, regular or diet pack, white or yellow, drained solids, 1/2 cup.	4%	65	6	70
Corn and peppers, canned, 1/2 cup.	4%	80	2	90
Corn, scalloped, frozen, 3-1/2 oz.	8%	60	50	140
Corn, white, frozen in butter sauce, 3-1/2 oz.	4%	60	25	90
Corn and peas with tomatoes, frozen, 3-1/2 oz.	4%	70	4	70
Corn flour, 1 cup.	14%	360	30	430
Corn fritters, 2″ diam., 1-1/2″ thick.	4%	55	70	130
Corn grits, degermed, cooked, enriched or unenriched, 1 cup.	4%	110	2	120
Corn flakes, ready-to-eat cereal with sugar incorporated, 1 cup.	4%	90	–	100
Corn flakes, sugar coated, 1 cup.	2%	150	–	150

*See note, p. 46.

	Protein* (% of U.S. RDA)	Carbohydrate Calories	Fat Calories	Total Calories
Corn, puffed cereal, pre-sweetened, 1 cup.	2%	110	–	110
Corn, puffed cereal, cocoa or fruit flavor, 1 cup.	2%	100	6	120
Corn pudding (milk recipe), 1 cup.	20%	130	100	260
Cornbread, home recipe, degermed cornmeal, piece 2-1/2" × 2-1/2" × 1-1/2".	10%	120	45	190
Cornbread, made from mix, 1 piece as above.	6%	110	50	180
Corn meal, degermed, enriched, or unenriched, dry form, 1 cup.	16%	430	15	500
Corn meal, self rising, no flour added, 1 cup.	18%	380	40	470
Corn meal, self rising, degermed, with or without added flour, 1 cup.	16%	420	15	490
Cornstarch, 1 tbsp.	–	30	–	30
Cottage cheese. (See cheeses.)				
Cottage pudding. (See cakes.)				
Cowpeas (blackeye peas), fresh, frozen, or canned, cooked, drained, 1/2 cup.	10%	60	6	90
Crab, including blue, dungeness, rock, king, cooked pieces of meat, 1 cup packed, about 1/3 lb.	60%	4	25	140
Crab, canned, drained, 1 cup, packed, about 1/3 lb.	60%	8	35	160

*See note, p. 46.

	Protein* (% of U.S. RDA)	Carbohydrate Calories	Fat Calories	Total Calories
Crab, deviled (made with bread, butter, eggs, catsup, etc.), 1 cup, about 1/2 lb.	60%	130	200	450
Crab, imperial (made with butter, flour, milk, eggs, seasonings, etc.), 1 cup, slightly less than 1/2 lb.	70%	35	150	320
Crackers, animal, about 175 per lb., 10 crackers.	2%	80	20	110
Crackers, cheese, 1" square, 420 per lb., 10 crackers.	2%	25	20	50
Crackers, graham, chocolate coated, about 2-1/2" square, 1 cracker, 1/2 oz.	–	35	30	60
Crackers, graham, sugar honey, 2-1/2" square, 1 cracker.	–	20	8	30
Crackers, saltines, about 2" square, 160 per lb., 1 cracker.	–	8	4	12
Crackers, cheese-peanut butter sandwiches, about 1-1/2" square, 1 sandwich.	2	8	4	15
Crackers, soda, biscuit-type, about 2-1/4" square, about 90 per lb., 1 biscuit.	–	15	6	22
Crackers, soup or oyster, about 550 per lb., 10 crackers.	–	20	10	30

*See note, p. 46.

	Protein* (% of U.S. RDA)	Carbohydrate Calories	Fat Calories	Total Calories
Cranberry juice cocktail (about 1/3 juice, sweetened with sugar), 6 oz. glass.	–	130	2	130
Cranberry sauce, canned, strained, 1/2 cup.	–	210	2	210
Cranberry sauce, homemade, unstrained, 1/2 cup.	–	250	2	250
Cranberry-orange relish, uncooked, 1/2 cup.	–	250	4	250
Cream, half-and-half, 1 tbsp.	2%	2	15	20
Cream, light coffee or table, 1 tbsp.	2%	2	30	30
Cream, light whipping or whipping, 1 tbsp.	–	2	40	45
Cream, heavy or heavy whipping, 1 tbsp.	–	2	50	55
Creamer, non-dairy, 1 tsp.	–	4	10	15
Cream puff, 1 custard filled, round, about 3-1/2" diameter × 2" thick.	15%	110	160	300
Cucumbers, raw, 6 slices 1/8" thick from 8" cucumber.	–	4	–	4
Cucumber pickles. (See pickles.)				
Custard, baked, 1/2 cup.	15%	60	7	150
Custard, frozen. (See ice cream.)				
Dandelion greens, boiled, 2/3 cup.	2%	20	1	25
Danish pastry. (See rolls.)				
Dates, whole, 1 date, pitted.	–	25	–	25
Dewberries. (See blackberries.)				

*See note, p. 46.

	Protein* (% of U.S. RDA)	Carbohydrate Calories	Fat Calories	Total Calories
Doughnut** cake-type, about 3-1/2".	4%	100	80	190
Doughnut** cake-type, about 1-1/2".	–	30	25	60
Doughnut, raised (yeast-leavened), about 3-3/4" diameter, plain.	4%	60	100	180
Eclair, custard-filled, chocolate iced, about 5" × 2".	10%	90	120	240
Egg, chicken, whole, fresh, boiled or poached, extra large size.	15%	2	60	90
Egg, chicken, whole, fresh, as above, large.	15%	2	50	80
Egg, chicken, whole, fresh, as above, medium.	12%	2	45	70
Egg, chicken, white of extra large egg.	10%	2	–	20
Egg, chicken, white of one large egg.	8%	2	–	18
Egg, chicken, white of one medium egg.	8%	–	–	15
Egg, chicken, yolk of extra-large egg.	6%	–	50	70
Egg, chicken, yolk of large egg.	6%	–	50	60
Egg, chicken, yolk of medium egg.	6%	–	40	50
Egg, chicken, fried, large.	15%	–	70	100
Egg, chicken, 1 large, scrambled.	15%	6	70	110

*See note, p. 46.
**Frostings and coatings add calories.

	Protein* (% of U.S. RDA)	Carbohydrate Calories	Fat Calories	Total Calories
Egg, duck, whole, fresh, boiled, etc.	20%	2	90	130
Egg omelet, using 2 large eggs.	30%	12	150	220
Egg rolls, frozen, 3-1/2 oz.	15%	130	50	200
Eggplant, cooked, diced, 1 cup.	4%	35	4	40
Eggplant, fried, frozen, 3-1/2 oz.	6%	100	170	290
Eggplant, Parmesan, frozen, 3-1/2 oz.	8%	60	100	200
Enchilada, beef and sauce, frozen, 6 oz. bag.	15%	120	110	260
Enchilada, cheese, frozen dinner, 12 oz.	35%	240	150	460
Endive, curly and escarole, raw, 1 cup.	2%	8	–	10
Farina, enriched and unenriched, cooked, regular and quick-cooking, 1 cup.	4%	90	2	110
Fats, cooking, various shortenings, 1 tbsp.	–	–	110	110
Fig, 1 fresh, medium, about 9 per lb.	–	40	2	40
Figs, canned, water pack, no added sweetener, 3 figs and 1-3/4 tbsp. liquid.	–	40	2	40
Figs, canned in heavy syrup, as above.	–	70	2	80
Filberts (hazelnuts), 10 shelled nuts.	2%	10	80	90
Fishcakes. (See codfish cakes.)				

*See note, p. 46.

	Protein* (% of U.S. RDA)	Carbohydrate Calories	Fat Calories	Total Calories
Fish dinner, frozen, about 9 oz.	40%	170	120	380
Fish and chips, frozen, 10 oz. plate.	50%	160	180	450
Fish loaf, cooked, 1 slice, about 5 oz.	50%	40	50	190
Fish sticks, frozen, breaded, cooked, about 4" × 1" × 1/2", 1 stick.	10%	8	25	50
Flounder, fillet, baked with butter or margarine, about 3.5 oz., 8" × 3" × 1/4".	70%	–	70	200
Flours. (See wheat, corn, etc.)				
Frankfurters. (See sausages.)				
Frostings. (See cake icings.)				
Frozen custard. (See ice cream.)				
Fruit-flavored beverages, carbonated, 12 oz. can or bottle (such as citrus flavors, cherry, grape, Tom Collins, etc.).	–	170	–	170
Fruit cocktail, canned, water pack, no sugar added, 1/2 cup.	1%	50	–	50
Fruit cocktail, canned, in heavy syrup, 1/2 cup.	1%	100	–	100
Fruit drinks. (See fruit types.)				
Garbanzos. (See chickpeas.)				
Garlic, raw, 1 clove, about 1-1/4" by 1/2".	–	4	–	4
Gefilte fish, canned or jarred, 3-1/2 oz.	20%	15	15	60

*See note, p. 46.

	Protein* (% of U.S. RDA)	Carbohydrate Calories	Fat Calories	Total Calories
Gelatin desserts made from powder, 1/2 cup.	**	70	–	70
Ginger ale, 12 oz. bottle or can.	–	120	–	120
Gingerbread. (See cakes.)				
Ginger, candied. (See candied ginger root.)				
Ginger root, fresh, 1 oz.	–	10	2	12
Gizzard, chicken, cooked, 1/2 cup diced, about 1/6 lb.	45%	2	20	110
Gizzard, turkey, cooked, 1/2 cup diced, about 1/6 lb.	45%	4	60	140
Goat's milk. (See milk.)				
Goose, roasted, 3 oz. serving.	60%	–	70	200
Gooseberries, fresh, 1/2 cup.	1%	30	2	30
Granadilla, purple (passion fruit), 1 fruit, about 12 per lb.	1%	15	2	15
Grapefruit, fresh, 1/2, all varieties and colors, about 3-1/2" diameter.	1%	40	2	45
Grapefruit juice, 6 oz. glass, unsweetened.	2%	70	2	80
Grapefruit juice, sweetened with sugar, 6 oz. glass.	2%	100	2	100
Grapefruit, canned sections, water pack, no sugar added, 1/2 cup.	1%	40	–	45

*See note, p. 46.
**Gelatins offer some protein, but of such low quality that it is not scored under the U.S. RDA system.

	Protein* (% of U.S. RDA)	Carbohydrate Calories	Fat Calories	Total Calories
Grapefruit, canned in heavy syrup, 1/2 cup.	1%	90	–	90
Grapefruit and orange juice, canned, or from concentrate, unsweetened, 6 oz. glass.	2%	75	2	80
Grapefruit and orange juice, canned, sugar added, 6 oz. glass.	2%	90	2	90
Grapefruit peel, candied. (See candied grapefruit.)				
Grapes, American slip-skin types, such as Concord, Delaware, Catawba, Niagara and Scuppernong, 1 cup, about 38 grapes.	2%	60	10	70
Grapes, European adherent-skin types, as Thompson Seedless, Emperor, Flame Tokay, Ribier, Muscat, Malaga, 1 cup, about 32 grapes.	2%	110	4	110
Grapes, canned, Thompson Seedless, packed in water, no added sugar, 1/2 cup.	–	70	–	70
Grapes, canned, Thompson Seedless, in heavy syrup, 1/2 cup.	–	100	2	100
Grape juice, canned or bottled, 6 oz. glass.	–	130	–	130
Grape juice, from frozen concentrate, 6 oz. glass.	–	100	–	100

*See note, p. 46.

	Protein * (% of U.S. RDA)	Carbohydrate Calories	Fat Calories	Total Calories
Grape drink, canned, 30% grape juice, 6 oz. glass.	–	100	–	100
Griddlecakes. (See pancakes.)				
Grits. (See corn grits.)				
Groundcherries (poha or cape gooseberries), raw, without husks, 1 cup.	4%	60	10	70
Haddock, fried, 1 fillet, about 6-1/2" × 2-1/2" × 5/8", 4 oz.	50%	25	60	180
Halibut, steak, Atlantic or Pacific, broiled, 1 piece, with butter or margarine, about 6-1/2" × 2-1/2" × 5/8", 4 oz.	70%	–	80	210
Ham. (See pork.)				
Hamburger. (See beef, ground.)				
Hazelnuts. (See filberts.)				
Headcheese. (See luncheon meat.)				
Heart, beef, lean, braised, about 1/3 lb.	100%	4	70	270
Heart, calf, braised, about 1/3 lb.	90%	10	120	300
Heart, chicken, cooked, about 1/3 lb.	80%	–	90	250
Heart, pork, cooked, 1/3 lb.	100%	2	90	280
Heart, lamb, cooked, 1/3 lb.	100%	6	190	380
Heart, turkey, cooked, 1/3 lb.	70%	2	170	310
Herring, canned, plain, 1 piece, about 3-1/2" × 2" × 3/4", about 3 oz.	50%	–	130	220

*See note, p. 46.

	Protein* (% of U.S. RDA)	Carbohydrate Calories	Fat Calories	Total Calories
Herring in tomato sauce, 2 pieces, about 2-1/2" × 1" × 3/4", about 3 oz.	30%	12	80	150
Herring, pickled, Bismarck, 2 pieces about 5" × 1-1/2" × 1/2", 3 oz.	35%	–	100	170
Herring, pickled, 6 marinated pieces, 1-3/4" × 1" × 1/2", about 3 oz.	40%	–	120	180
Honey, 1 tbsp.	–	70	–	70
Honeydew melon, wedge, 7" long × 2" wide at center.	2%	45	4	50
Horseradish, prepared, 1 tsp.	–	2	–	2
Ice cream, regular, 10% fat, 1 cup.	15%	110	130	260
Ice cream, rich, 16% fat, 1 cup.	8%	110	210	330
Ice cream, soft serve (frozen custard), 1 cup.	15%	140	160	330
Ice milk (5.1% fat), 1 cup.	20%	160	80	270
Ice milk (soft, custard type), 1 cup.	8%	110	210	330
Ices, water, lime or other flavors.	2%	250	–	250
Icings. (See cake icings.)				
Jams, made with nutritive sweetener, 1 tbsp.	–	60	–	60
Jellies, made with nutritive sweetener, 1 tbsp.	–	50	–	50
Kale, leaves, cooked, drained, 1 cup.	8%	25	8	40
Kidney, beef, cooked, about 1/3 lb.	100%	4	150	350

*See note, p. 46.

	Protein* (% of U.S. RDA)	Carbohydrate Calories	Fat Calories	Total Calories
Knockwurst. (See sausages.)				
Kohlrabi, boiled, 1 cup.	4%	35	2	40
Kumquat, 1 raw.	–	12	–	12
Lamb leg, roasted, 2 pieces, about 4" × 2-1/4" × 1/4", lean with fat, about 3 oz.	50%	–	140	240
Lamb leg, as above, but fat trimmed, 2 pieces, 3 oz.	50%	–	50	160
Lamb, loin chops, broiled, lean with fat, about 1/3 lb., 1 chop.	45%	–	250	340
Lamb, loin chops, broiled, fat trimmed, 1 chop, 1/3 lb.	40%	–	40	120
Lamb, rib chops, broiled, lean with fat, 1 chop, about 1/3 lb.	40%	–	290	360
Lamb, rib chops, broiled, fat trimmed, 1 chop, 1/3 lb.	35%	–	50	120
Lamb shoulder, roasted, lean with fat, 3 pieces, each 2-1/2" square × 1/4" thick, about 3 oz.	40%	–	210	290
Lamb shoulder, as above, but fat trimmed.	50%	–	80	170
Lard, 1 tbsp.	–	–	120	120
Lasagna, frozen, 8 oz.	40%	90	230	410
Lemon, wedge, 1/4 medium fruit, 1 oz.	–	6	–	6
Lemon juice, fresh, 1 tbsp., 1/2 oz.	–	4	–	4

*See note, p. 46.

	Protein* (% of U.S. RDA)	Carbohydrate Calories	Fat Calories	Total Calories
Lemon juice, canned or frozen, unsweetened, 1 tbsp.	–	4	–	4
Lemon peel, raw grated, 1 tsp.	–	2	–	2
Lemonade, from frozen concentrate, 1 cup.	–	110	–	110
Lentils, cooked, 1/2 cup.	12%	80	–	110
Lettuce, raw, butterhead, loose leaf, bunching, and Romain varieties, 1 cup chopped or shredded pieces.	–	8	2	10
Lettuce, raw, crisphead varieties, such as Iceberg, New York, Great Lakes, 1 cup of pieces.	–	8	–	10
Lima beans. (See beans.)				
Lime, pulp of 3 oz. fruit.	–	25	–	25
Lime juice, fresh or canned, 1 tbsp.	–	6	–	6
Limeade, from frozen concentrate, 1 cup.	–	110	–	110
Liver, beef, fried, slice about 6-1/2" × 2-1/2" × 3/8", about 3 oz. when cooked.	50%	20	80	200
Liver, calf, fried, slice as above.	60%	15	100	220
Liver, chicken, 3 whole, about 3 oz.	50%	10	35	210
Liver, chicken, chopped, 1/2 cup.	40%	8	30	120
Liver, pork, about 1/3 lb.	60%	8	90	210
Liver, lamb, about 3 oz.	60%	10	100	230

*See note, p. 46.

	Protein* (% of U.S. RDA)	Carbohydrate Calories	Fat Calories	Total Calories
Liver, turkey, chopped, 1/2 cup, 2-1/2 oz.	45%	8	30	120
Liver paste. (See pâté.)				
Liverwurst, or sausage. (See sausage.)				
Lobster, cooked northern, 1 cup pieces, about 1/3 lb. meat.	60%	2	20	140
Lobster newburg, 1 cup.	100%	50	250	490
Lobster paste. (See shrimp paste.)				
Loganberries, raw, 1 cup.	2%	90	8	100
Loquats, raw, 10 fruits, 1/3 lb.	–	60	2	60
Luncheon meat, canned deviled ham, 1 oz., about 2 tbsp.	8%	–	80	100
Luncheon meat, boiled ham, 1 oz.	10%	–	45	70
Luncheon meat, headcheese, 1 oz.	10%	25	40	80
Luncheon meat, pork, cured ham or shoulder, chopped, spiced or unspiced, canned, 1 oz.	10%	2	60	80
Luncheon meat, meatloaf, 1 oz.	10%	4	35	60
Luncheon meat, minced ham, 1 oz.	8%	6	45	60
Luncheon meat, potted meat (includes beef, chicken, turkey), canned, 1 oz., about 2 tbsp.	10%	–	50	70

*See note, p. 46.

	Protein* (% of U.S. RDA)	Carbohydrate Calories	Fat Calories	Total Calories
Luncheon meat, scrapple, slice of prepackaged loaf, about 2-1/2" square, 1/4" thick, about 1 oz.	6%	15	35	60
Luncheon meat, souse, prepackaged slice, 1 oz., 3-7/8" square and 1/8" thick.	8%	2	35	50
Lychee nuts, raw, 10.	2%	60	2	65
Macaroni, cooked lengths, elbows or shells, 1 cup.	8%	130	6	160
Macaroni and cheese, home recipe, 1 cup.	30%	160	200	430
Macaroni and cheese, canned, 1 cup.	15%	100	90	230
Macaroni and beef dinner, frozen, 11-12 oz.	20%	220	140	400
Macaroni and cheese entrée, frozen, 8 oz.	25%	130	110	300
Mackerel, Atlantic, broiled with fat, 1 fillet, about 4 oz.	50%	–	150	250
Mackerel, Pacific, canned, about 1/3 can, approx. 5 oz.	70%	–	130	260
Mackerel, salted, fillet, 7-3/4" × 2-1/2" × 1/2", about 4 oz.	45%	–	250	340
Mandarin oranges. (See tangerines.)				
Mangos, raw, 1 whole fruit.	2%	160	8	160

*See note, p. 46.

	Protein* (% of U.S. RDA)	Carbohydrate Calories	Fat Calories	Total Calories
Margarine, regular type, 1 tbsp.	–	–	100	100
Margarine, whipped type, about 1/8 stick, 1 tbsp.	–	–	70	70
Margarine, diet type, 1 tbsp.	–	–	50	50
Marmalade, citrus, 1 tbsp.	–	60	–	60
Mexican dinner, frozen, 16-18 oz.	40%	290	240	650
Meat loaf, frozen dinner, 11 oz.	40%	120	200	410
Meat loaf. (See lunch meat.)				
Milk, cow, whole, 1 cup.	20%	50	80	160
Milk, cow, lowfat, 2% nonfat milk solids added, 1 cup.	25%	60	45	150
Milk, skim, (nonfat), 1 cup.	20%	50	2	90
Milk, canned, evaporated, 1 cup.	40%	100	180	350
Milk, condensed, sweetened, 1 cup.	60%	670	240	980
Milk, dry, regular whole, 1 cup.	70%	200	330	640
Milk, dry, nonfat regular, 1 cup.	100%	250	10	440
Milk, dry, nonfat instant, 1 cup.	50%	140	4	240
Milk, malted, powder, 3 heaping tsp.	6%	80	20	120
Milk, with chocolate, made with skim milk, 1 cup.	20%	110	50	190
Milk, with chocolate, made with whole milk, 1 cup.	20%	110	80	210
Milk, hot chocolate or cocoa, 1 cup.	20%	100	110	240

*See note, p. 46.

	Protein* (% of U.S. RDA)	Carbohydrate Calories	Fat Calories	Total Calories
Milk, goat, 1 cup.	15%	45	70	160
Molasses, cane, first extraction, 1 tbsp.	–	50	–	50
Mortadella. (See sausage.)				
Muffin, home recipe, plain, 1 muffin.	4%	70	35	120
Muffin, blueberry, or bran, 1 muffin.	4%	70	35	110
Muffin, corn, 1 muffin.	4%	80	35	130
Muffins, corn, from mix, 1 muffin.	4%	80	40	130
Mushrooms, raw, 1/2 cup.	2%	20	4	25
Mushrooms, frozen in butter, 3-1/2 oz.	2%	10	30	60
Muskmelon. (See canteloup.)				
Mustard greens, cooked, 1 cup.	4%	20	6	30
Mustard spinach, cooked, 1 cup.	4%	20	4	30
Mustard, prepared, brown, 1 tsp.	–	2	2	5
Mustard, prepared, yellow, 1 tsp.	–	2	2	4
Nectarine, raw, 1 fruit, 2-1/2" diam.	2%	90	–	90
Noodles, egg, enriched, cooked, 1 cup.	10%	150	20	200
Noodles, chow mein, canned, 1 cup.	10%	100	100	220
Nuts. (See varieties.)				
Oat flakes, instant-cooking, cooked, 1 cup.	10%	125	15	170
Oat granules, flavored, cooked, 1 cup.	8%	110	15	150

*See note, p. 46.

	Protein* (% of U.S. RDA)	Carbohydrate Calories	Fat Calories	Total Calories
Oatmeal (or rolled oats), regular or quick-cooking, cooked, 1 cup.	8%	90	20	130
Oat and wheat cereal, cooked, 1 cup.	10%	120	20	160
Oat cereal, ready-to-eat, shredded, added protein, sugar, 1 cup, dry.	15%	130	8	170
Oat cereal, ready-to-eat, puffed, added sugar, 1 cup, dry.	4%	80	15	100
Oat and corn cereal, puffed, sugar-coated, 1 cup, dry.	4%	120	10	140
Ocean perch (redfish), Atlantic, fresh, fried, 1 fillet about 7" × 1-3/4" × 5/8", about 3 oz. cooked.	35%	25	100	190
Ocean perch (redfish), Atlantic, frozen, breaded, fried, reheated, 1 fillet, about 3 oz., as above.	35%	60	150	280
Oils, salad or cooking, including corn, safflower, cottonseed, soybean and cottonseed blend, soybean, olive, peanut, etc., 1 cup, average.	–	–	1920	1920
Oils, salad or cooking, as above, 1 tbsp., average.	–	–	120	120
Okra, boiled, slices, 2/3 cup.	4%	25	4	30
Okra, frozen, boiled, cuts, 2/3 cup.	4%	45	2	50

*See note, p. 46.

	Protein* (% of U.S. RDA)	Carbohydrate Calories	Fat Calories	Total Calories
Olives, green, pickled, 10 "large" size, about 98 per lb.	–	2	45	45
Olives, ripe, Ascolano or Manzanillo 10 "extra large" size, 82 per lb.	–	4	60	60
Olives, ripe, mission, 10 "extra large" size, 82 per lb.	–	6	90	90
Olives, ripe, Sevillano, 10 "giant" size, about 53–60 per lb.	2%	8	60	70
Olives, ripe, salt-cured, oil-coated, Greek style, 10 "extra large" size, about 137 per lb.	–	10	90	90
Onions, French fried, canned, 3-1/2 oz.	–	180	440	620
Onions, mature, 1 tbsp. chopped.	–	4	–	4
Onions, mature, 1/2 cup, chopped.	2%	30	–	35
Onions, young green, bunching type, 1 tbsp. chopped.	–	2	–	2
Onions, young green, bunching type, tops only, chopped, 1 tbsp.	–	2	–	2
Onions in cream sauce, frozen, 3-1/2 oz.	4%	30	8	45
Onion rings, fried, frozen, 3-1/2 oz.	8%	120	160	290

*See note, p. 46.

	Protein* (% of U.S. RDA)	Carbohydrate Calories	Fat Calories	Total Calories
Oranges, all California and Florida varieties, 1 medium orange, approx. 3″ diam.	2%	70	2	70
Oranges, mandarin, canned, 1/2 cup.	2%	80	–	80
Orange juice, fresh or canned, unsweetened, from California or Florida oranges, 6 oz. glass.	2%	80	4	90
Orange juice, canned, sugar added, 6 oz. glass.	2%	90	4	100
Orange juice from frozen concentrate, prepared, 6 oz. glass.	2%	90	2	90
Orange juice from dehydrated crystals, prepared, 6 oz. glass.	2%	80	4	90
Orange peel, raw, grated, 1 tbsp.	–	6	–	6
Orange peel, candied. (See candied.)				
Orange-grapefruit juice. (See grapefruit.)				
Orange-apricot drink, about 40% fruit juice, canned, 6 oz. glass.	–	90	2	90
Oysterplant. (See salsify.)				
Oysters, Eastern, raw or canned, meat only, about 10 large, 1/3 lb.	30%	20	25	100

*See note, p. 46.

	Protein* (% of U.S. RDA)	Carbohydrate Calories	Fat Calories	Total Calories
Oysters, Pacific, raw or canned, meat only, about 5 small, 1/3 lb.	35%	40	30	140
Oysters, fried, 4 oz., about 10.	20%	80	140	270
Oyster stew, home prepared, 1 part oysters to 2 parts milk, 1 cup.	30%	45	140	230
Pancake, home recipe, 6" diam.	10%	90	50	160
Pancake, plain or buttermilk, from mix, egg and milk added, 6" diam.	10%	90	50	160
Pancake, buckwheat and other cereal flours, from mix, egg and milk added, 6" diam.	10%	70	60	150
Papaya, raw, 1/2 of 1 fruit, about 5" × 3-1/2".	2%	60	2	60
Parsley, raw, chopped, 1 tbsp.	–	2	–	2
Parsnip, fresh, cooked, cut up, 1 cup, (equals 1 large parsnip, 9" long.)	4%	90	8	100
Passion fruit. (See granadilla.)				
Pastry, frozen, typical, 1/8 of round cake.	4%	80	80	170
Pastry shell. (See pie crust.)				
Pâté de foie gras, canned, 1 tbsp., about 1/2 oz.	4%	2	50	60

*See note, p. 46.

	Protein* (% of U.S. RDA)	Carbohydrate Calories	Fat Calories	Total Calories
Pawpaw, common North American type, raw, 1 fruit, 3-3/4″ × 2″, about 4-1/2 oz.	8%	70	8	80
Peaches, 1 raw, 2-3/4″ diam., about 2-1/2 per lb.	2%	60	2	60
Peaches, canned halves, water pack, no sugar added, 2 halves with 4 tbsp. liquid.	2%	60	2	60
Peaches, canned clingstone or freestone, in heavy syrup, 2 halves with about 4 tbsp. liquid.	2%	150	2	150
Peaches, canned clingstone or freestone, slices in water pack, no added sugar, 1/2 cup.	–	40	–	40
Peaches, canned clingstone or freestone, slices in heavy syrup, 1/2 cup.	–	100	2	100
Peaches, dried, halves, 2 large halves.	2%	80	2	80
Peaches, frozen slices, sugar added, thawed fruit and syrup, 1/2 cup.	–	110	2	110
Peaches, spiced, canned, 1/2 cup.	–	120	–	120
Peach nectar, canned, 6 oz. glass.	–	90	–	90
Peanuts, roasted in shell, 10 jumbo nuts, about 1 oz.	8%	15	80	110

*See note, p. 46.

	Protein* (% of U.S. RDA)	Carbohydrate Calories	Fat Calories	Total Calories
Peanuts, shelled, roasted, salted, 1 tbsp. chopped, 20 Spanish, or 10 Virginia.	4%	6	40	50
Peanut butter, small amounts of fat and sugar added, 1 tbsp.	6%	10	70	90
Peanut butter, no fat or sugar added, 1 tbsp.	6%	10	60	80
Peanut flour, defatted, 1 cup.	40%	80	50	220
Peanut oil. (See oils.)				
Pear, 1 whole raw, Bartlett, 3-1/2" × 2-1/2", 2-1/2 per lb.	2%	100	6	100
Pear, whole raw, Bosc, 3" × 2-1/2", 3 per lb.	2%	90	6	90
Pear, whole raw, D'Anjou, 3-1/2" × 3", 2 per lb.	2%	120	8	120
Pear, canned, water pack, no added sugar, 2 halves, 2 tbsp. liquid.	–	30	2	30
Pear, canned, heavy syrup, 2 halves, 2 tbsp. syrup.	–	80	2	80
Pear, dried, sulphured, 2 halves.	2%	90	6	90
Pear nectar, 40% fruit juice, 6 oz. glass.	–	100	4	100
Peas, black eye, frozen, 1/2 cup.	10%	60	2	90
Peas in cream sauce, frozen, 3-1/2 oz.	6%	40	8	70

*See note, p. 46.

	Protein* (% of U.S. RDA)	Carbohydrate Calories	Fat Calories	Total Calories
Peas, green, canned, sweet, (sweet wrinkled peas, sugar peas), 2/3 cup, drained.	8%	70	4	90
Peas, fresh or frozen, cooked, 2/3 cup.	8%	50	4	70
Peas, frozen in butter sauce, 3-1/2 oz.	6%	40	25	80
Peas and carrots, frozen, cooked, 2/3 cup.	6%	45	4	60
Peas, dry, mature seeds, split, cooked, 2/3 cup.	15%	110	4	150
Pecans, 10 shelled halves, jumbo size, 1/2 oz.	2%	8	90	100
Pecans, chopped or pieces, 1/2 cup.	8%	35	380	410
Peppers, hot chili, immature green, canned, chili sauce, 1/2 cup.	2%	25	–	25
Peppers, hot chili, mature red, canned, chili sauce, 1/2 cup.	2%	20	6	25
Pepper, hot chili, red, dry powder, 1 tbsp., added seasoning (chili powder).	2%	15	6	20
Pepper, sweet green, raw, or cooked, 1 pepper, 3-3/4" × 3", 2-1/4 per lb.	4%	30	2	35
Pepper, green, raw, chopped, 1 cup.	2%	30	2	35
Pepper, red, mature, raw, as above.	4%	45	4	50

*See note, p. 46

	Protein* (% of U.S. RDA)	Carbohydrate Calories	Fat Calories	Total Calories
Persimmon, raw, whole, Japanese, 3" × 2-1/2", 2-1/4 per lb.	2%	130	6	130
Persimmon, native, raw, whole, 1 oz.	–	35	–	35
Pickle, dill, cucumber, whole medium, about 3-3/4" × 1-1/4" diam., 2 oz.	–	6	–	7
Pickle, bread and butter or fresh, sugar added, 1/4" slices, 1/3 cup, about 2 oz.	–	40	8	45
Pickle, sour, whole, 3-3/4" × 1-1/4" (medium), about 2 oz.	–	6	–	7
Pickle, sweet, gherkins, small, 2-1/2" × 3/4", 4 pickles, 2 oz.	–	90	4	90
Pickle, chowchow or mustard (added cauliflower, onion, mustard), sour, 1/4 cup, about 2 oz.	2%	10	6	20
Pickle, chowchow or mustard, sweet, as above, but added sugar, 1/4 cup, about 2 oz.	2%	70	4	70
PIES: *All servings shown are wedges cut from 9" pies. A wedge is one eighth of pie.*				
Pie, apple.	4%	180	120	300
Pie, banana custard.	10%	140	100	250
Pie, blackberry or blueberry.	4%	160	120	290

*See note, p. 46.

	Protein* (% of U.S. RDA)	Carbohydrate Calories	Fat Calories	Total Calories
Pie, Boston cream. (See cakes.)				
Pie, butterscotch.	8%	170	110	300
Pie, cherry.	4%	180	120	310
Pie, chocolate chiffon.	10%	140	110	270
Pie, chocolate meringue.	10%	150	120	290
Pie, coconut custard.	15%	110	130	270
Pie, custard.	15%	110	110	250
Pie, lemon chiffon.	10%	140	90	250
Pie, lemon meringue.	8%	160	100	270
Pie, mince.	4%	190	120	320
Pie, peach.	4%	180	110	300
Pie, pecan.	10%	210	210	430
Pie, pineapple.	4%	180	110	300
Pie, pineapple chiffon or custard.	10%	130	90	230
Pie, pumpkin or sweet potato.	8%	110	120	240
Pie, raisin.	4%	200	110	320
Pie, rhubarb.	4%	180	110	300
Pie, strawberry.	2%	110	70	180
FROZEN PIES: *8" in diameter, (1/8 wedges are smaller).*				
Pie, frozen, apple, baked.	2%	110	60	170
Pie, frozen, cherry, baked.	2%	130	80	210
Pie, frozen, coconut custard.	8%	90	80	190
Pie, from mixes, filling and crust, coconut custard, 1/8 wedge of 8" pie, egg yolks and milk added.	8%	120	70	200
Piecrust, homemade, 1 pie shell.	15%	320	540	900

*See note, p. 46.

	Protein* (% of U.S. RDA)	Carbohydrate Calories	Fat Calories	Total Calories
Piecrust, from mix, 1 pie shell.	20%	340	500	890
Pigs' feet, pickled, 2 oz.	20%	–	80	110
Pimientos, canned, 1 2-oz. jar.	–	15	2	15
Pineapple, raw, 1 slice, 3-1/2" × 3/4", about 3 oz.	–	50	2	50
Pineapple, candied. (See candied.)				
Pineapple, canned in water no added sugar, 1/2 cup, about 4 oz.	–	50	–	50
Pineapple, canned in heavy syrup, 1/2 cup of cuts, about 4-1/2 oz.	–	100	2	100
Pineapple, canned in heavy syrup, 1 large slice, 3-1/2" diam., 8 chunks or 17 tidbits, with syrup, 3.7 oz.	–	80	–	80
Pineapple, canned in extra heavy syrup, 3.7 oz. serving as above.	–	100	–	100
Pineapple, frozen chunks, sugar added, 1/2 cup, about 4.3 oz.	–	110	2	110
Pineapple juice, reconstituted from frozen or canned, unsweetened, 6-oz. glass.	–	100	–	100
Pineapple and grapefruit juice drink, about 50% juices, 6-oz. glass.	–	100	–	100

*See note, p. 46.

	Protein* (% of U.S. RDA)	Carbohydrate Calories	Fat Calories	Total Calories
Pineapple and grapefruit juice drink, about 40% juices, 6-oz. glass.	–	100	2	100
Pine nuts, pignolias, shelled, 1 oz.	15%	15	120	160
Pine nuts, piñon, shelled, 1 oz.	6%	25	150	180
Pistachio nuts, 2 oz. in shell or 1 oz. shelled.	8%	20	140	170
Pitanga (Surinam cherry), 2 raw fruits, about 1/2 oz.	–	4	–	5
Pizza, cheese, homemade style, wedge, 1/8 of 14" pizza.	15%	70	50	150
Pizza, sausage, homemade style, wedge, 1/8 of 14" pizza.	10%	80	60	160
Pizza, cheese, commercial frozen, baked, 1/7 of 10" pizza.	10%	80	40	140
Plantain, (baking banana) about 11" × 2", 13 oz.	4%	300	10	310
Plum, damson, raw, 2 1" plums.	–	15	–	15
Plum, Japanese and hybrid, 1 plum, 2-1/8" diam.	–	30	–	30
Plum, prune type, raw, 1 plum, 1-1/2" diam.	–	20	–	20
Plums, canned, purple, in water, no sugar added, 3 plums and 2 tbsp. liquid.	–	50	2	50

*See note, p. 46.

	Protein* (% of U.S. RDA)	Carbohydrate Calories	Fat Calories	Total Calories
Plums, canned, purple, in heavy syrup, 3 plums and 2-3/4 tbsp. liquid.	–	110	–	110
Pokeberry (poke) shoots, cooked, drained, 1 cup.	6%	20	6	30
Pollock, cooked, creamed, 1 cup.	80%	40	130	320
Pomegranate, raw, 3-3/8" diam., 2-3/4" high, about 10 oz.	2%	100	4	100
Popcorn, plain, 1 cup popped.	2%	20	2	25
Popcorn, "buttered" with fat, 1 cup.	2%	20	20	40
Popcorn, sugar coated (or caramel), 1 cup.	4%	120	10	134
Popover, home recipe, 2-3/4" diam.	6%	40	35	90
Pork, leg, baked or roasted, lean with fat, 2 pieces, 4" × 2-1/4" × 1/4", 3 oz.	45%	–	230	320
Pork, leg, baked or roasted, as above, but fat trimmed.	60%	–	80	180
Pork loin or loin chops, baked or roasted, lean with fat, 2 pieces, each about 2-1/2" square and 3/4" thick, 6 oz., boned.	90%	–	440	620

*See note, p. 46.

	Protein* (% of U.S. RDA)	Carbohydrate Calories	Fat Calories	Total Calories
Pork loin or loin chops, 2 pieces as above, 6 oz. boned, fat trimmed.	110%	–	220	430
Pork, loin chops, broiled, 2 chops cut 3 per pound (yielding 2.7 oz. of boneless meat each), lean with fat.	90%	–	440	610
Pork, loin chops, broiled, 2 chops as above, but fat trimmed.	80%	–	150	300
Pork, shoulder cut, Boston butt, fat trimmed, roasted, pieces 2-1/2" square, 1/2" thick, boneless, 6 oz.	100%	–	220	410
Pork, shoulder cut, picnic, fat trimmed, roasted or simmered, pieces without bone, 2-1/2" square, 1/2" thick, 3 pieces, 6 oz.	110%	–	150	360
Pork, spareribs, cooked, lean with fat, 6.3 oz. of meat, yield from 1 lb. of ribs.	80%	–	630	790
Pork, cured, ham, baked or roasted, 2 pieces, about 4" × 2-1/4" × 1/2", 6 oz., fat trimmed.	100%	–	140	320
Pork, cured, Boston butt, 3 pieces 2-1/2" square, 1/2" thick, fat trimmed, meat only, 6 oz.	100%	–	210	410

*See note, p. 46.

	Protein* (% of U.S. RDA)	Carbohydrate Calories	Fat Calories	Total Calories
Pork, cured, picnic ham, baked, fat trimmed, meat only, 2-1/2" square, 1/2" thick, 3 pieces, 6 oz.	110%	–	150	360
Pork, cured, canned ham, baked, slice, about 1/3 pound, includes total contents of can.	60%	6	170	290
Pork, cured. (See also bacon.)				
Potato, baked or boiled in skin or peeled, long type, raw, 1 potato, 4-3/4" × 2-1/3", about 2 per lb.	6%	130	2	140
Potato, baked or boiled in skin, or peeled, round type, 2-1/2" diam., 2 per lb., raw.	4%	90	–	100
Potatoes, French fried, strips 3-1/2" to 4", 10 strips, less than 3 oz.	6%	110	90	210
Potatoes, French fried, frozen, heated, 10 strips 3-1/2" to 4".	4%	100	60	170
Potatoes, mashed, milk and butter, 1/2 cup.	4%	50	35	90
Potatoes, baked with cheese or sour cream, frozen, 3-1/2 oz.	6%	90	70	170
Potato chips, 10 chips, about 1-3/4" × 2-1/2", about 3/4 oz.	2%	40	70	110

*See note, p. 46.

	Protein* (% of U.S. RDA)	Carbohydrate Calories	Fat Calories	Total Calories
Potato salad, home recipe, made with salad dressing, 2/3 cup.	8%	110	40	170
Potato salad, home recipe, made with mayonnaise or French dressing, hard-cooked eggs, etc., 2/3 cup.	6%	90	140	240
Potato salad, canned, 5 oz.	4%	100	120	230
Potato sticks, 1 oz.	2%	60	90	150
Pretzels, twisted, about 2-3/4" diam., 1 pretzel.	2%	50	6	60
Pretzels, 10 rings, 1-1/2" diam.	4%	60	8	80
Pretzels, 10 logs, 3" × 1/2".	8%	150	20	200
Pretzels, 1 rod, 7-1/2" long, 1/2" diam.	2%	40	6	60
Pretzels, 10 sticks, about 3" × 1/8".	—	20	2	25
Prunes, dried, raw, 1/2 cup, 2 oz.	2%	180	2	180
Prunes, "softenized," raw, 1/2 cup, about 3 oz.	2%	220	4	220
Prunes, cooked, 1/2 cup, about 4-1/2 oz.	2%	130	2	130
Prunes, cooked, sugar added, 1/2 cup, about 5 oz.	2%	210	2	210
Prunes, canned, 1/2 cup.	2%	170	4	170
Prune juice, canned, 6 oz. glass.	2%	150	2	150
Prune whip, baked, served cold, about 4-1/2 oz., 1 cup.	8%	190	2	200

*See note, p. 46.

	Protein* (% of U.S. RDA)	Carbohydrate Calories	Fat Calories	Total Calories	
Pudding, home recipe, chocolate, 1 cup.	15%	270	120	390	
Pudding, home recipe, vanilla (blanc-mange), 1 cup.	15%	160	90	280	
Pudding, made from mix, with milk, 1 cup.	15%	240	70	320	
Pudding, made from mix, with milk, instant, no cooking, 1 cup.	15%	250	60	330	
Pumpkin, canned, 1 cup.	2%	40	—	40	
Pumpkin and squash seed kernels, 1/4 cup, 1-1/4 oz.	15%	20	150	190	
Rabbit, domestic, cooked, meat, 1 cup.	90%	—	130	300	
Radishes, raw, medium, 3/4" to 1" diam., 3 radishes, about 1/2 oz.	—	2	—	2	
Raisins, seedless, unbleached, raw, 1/2 oz. package, 1-1/2 tbsp.	—	45	—	45	
Raisins, 1/2 cup, not packed, about 5 oz.	6%	220	2	220	
Raspberries, raw, black, 1 cup.	2%	80	15	100	
Raspberries, raw, red, 1 cup.	2%	70	6	80	
Raspberries, canned, unsweetened, 1/2 cup.	2%	40	—	45	
Raspberries, frozen, sugar added, 1/2 cup.	2%	120	2	120	

*See note, p. 46.

	Protein* (% of U.S. RDA)	Carbohydrate Calories	Fat Calories	Total Calories
Ravioli, beef, canned in meat sauce, 7-1/2 oz.	20%	140	60	240
Ravioli, beef or cheese, frozen, 4 oz.	20%	150	50	260
Rhubarb, raw, cooked with sugar, 2/3 cup.	2%	190	2	190
Rhubarb, frozen, cooked with sugar, 1/2 cup.	2%	200	2	200
Rice, brown, cooked, 1 cup.	8%	200	10	230
Rice, white, long grain, polished, cooked, 1 cup.	6%	200	2	220
Rice, parboiled, long grain, cooked, 1 cup.	6%	160	2	190
Rice, white instant, pre-cooked, long grain, 1 cup.	6%	200	–	220
Rice, mixed or wild with brown or white, 1 cup.	8%	160	2	200
Rice, cooked cereal, granulated, 1 cup.	4%	110	–	120
Rice cereal, puffed, with sugar, 1 cup.	2%	110	–	120
Rice cereal, puffed, no sugar added, 1 cup.	2%	50	–	60
Rice cereal, puffed with honey or cocoa, 1 cup.	2%	120	15	140
Rice cereal, shredded, added sugar, 1 cup.	2%	90	–	100
Rice cereal, protein and sugar added, 1 cup.	6%	60	–	80
Rice pudding with raisins, 1/2 cup.	8%	140	35	190

*See note, p. 46.

	Protein* (% of U.S. RDA)	Carbohydrate Calories	Fat Calories	Total Calories
Rock cornish game hen, 1 hen, 9–10 oz.	110%	–	300	500
Rockfish, oven steamed, 1 fillet, 7" × 3-3/8" × 5/8", about 4 oz.	45%	8	25	120
Roe, herring, canned, 1 oz.	15%	4	8	35
Roll, cloverleaf, from home-type recipe, 2-1/2" × 2", about 1-1/4 oz.	4%	80	25	120
Roll, Danish pastry, plain, no fruit or nuts, wedge, 1/8 of 8" cake, 1-1/2 oz.	4%	80	90	180
Roll, Danish pastry, individual round, 4-1/4" diam., 1" thick, about 2-1/4 oz.	8%	120	140	270
Roll, hard, commercial, kaiser type, 3-3/4" diam., 2" thick, 1-3/4 oz.	8%	120	15	160
Roll, cloverleaf, commercial, or brown and serve, pull-aparts, 2" square, 1 oz.	4%	60	15	80
Roll, frankfurter or hamburger, 1-1/2 oz.	6%	80	20	120
Roll from frozen dough, parkerhouse, baked, 1 oz.	4%	50	15	80
Roll, from roll mix and water, baked, 1-1/4 oz.	4%	80	15	110

*See note, p. 46.

	Protein* (% of U.S. RDA)	Carbohydrate Calories	Fat Calories	Total Calories	
Roll, salt stick, 4-1/4″ × 1/2″, 3 sticks.	6%	90	8	120	
Roll, salt stick, Vienna bread type, stick 6-1/2″ × 1-1/4″.	6%	80	10	110	
Root beer, 12 oz. can or bottle.	–	150	–	150	
Rusk, Holland type, 3-3/8″ × 1/2″, about 1/3 oz.	2%	25	8	40	
Rutabagas, cubed, 2/3 cup, cooked.	2%	35	2	40	
Rye flour, light, unsifted, 1 cup.	15%	320	10	360	
Rye flour, dark, unsifted, 1 cup.	30%	350	30	420	
Rye wafers, whole grain, 4 wafers, about 3-1/2″ × 2″, 1 oz.	6%	80	2	90	
Safflower oil. (See oils.)					
Salad dressing, blue or Roquefort cheese, commercial, 1 tbsp.	2%	4	70	80	
Salad dressing, blue or Roquefort cheese, commercial, low fat, 1 tbsp.	2%	2	8	15	
Salad dressing, French, commercial, 1 tbsp.	–	10	60	70	
Salad dressing, French, low fat, 1 tbsp.	–	10	6	15	
Salad dressing, Italian, commercial, 1 tbsp.	–	4	80	80	

*See note, p. 46.

	Protein* (% of U.S. RDA)	Carbohydrate Calories	Fat Calories	Total Calories
Salad dressing, Italian, low fat, 1 tbsp.	—	2	6	8
Salad dressing, mayonnaise, commercial, 1 tbsp.	—	2	100	100
Salad dressing, mayonnaise type, 1 tbsp.	—	8	60	70
Salad dressing, mayonnaise type, low-cal., 1 tbsp.	—	4	20	20
Salad dressing, Russian, commercial, 1 tbsp.	—	6	70	80
Salad dressing, thousand island, commercial, 1 tbsp.	—	10	70	80
Salad dressing, thousand island, low-cal., 1 tbsp.	—	10	20	30
Salad dressing, French, home recipe, 1 tbsp.	—	2	90	90
Salad dressing, cooked, home recipe, 1 tbsp.	2%	10	15	25
Salami. (See sausage.)				
Salmon, canned Atlantic, 1/2 of 7-3/4 oz. can, about 3.8 oz.	50%	—	120	220
Salmon, canned Chinook, 1/2 of 7-3/4 oz. can, about 3.8 oz.	50%	—	140	230
Salmon, canned Chum, silver, pink, 1/2 of 7-3/4 oz. can, about 3.8 oz.	50%	—	70	170

*See note, p. 46.

	Protein* (% of U.S. RDA)	Carbohydrate Calories	Fat Calories	Total Calories
Salmon, canned sockeye, red, 1/2 of 7-3/4 oz. can, about 3.8 oz.	50%	–	90	190
Salmon, fresh, broiled or baked with butter, steak about 6-3/4" × 2-1/2" × 1", 5 oz.	80%	–	80	230
Salmon rice loaf, piece about 4" × 2-1/2" × 1-1/2", about 6 oz.	40%	50	70	210
Salmon, smoked (lox), 1 oz.	15%	–	25	50
Sandwich spread, canned, with pickle, 1/4 cup, for sandwich, 2.2 oz.	–	40	200	230
Salisbury steak, frozen dinner, 11 oz.	45%	100	230	400
Salisbury steak, frozen large dinner, 16 oz.	60%	220	270	620
Salsify, boiled, drained, pieces, 2/3 cup.	4%	50	8	70
Sardines, Atlantic, canned in oil, 3-3/4 oz., net from small can.	50%	–	90	190
Sardines, Norway, canned in oil, 3 oz., net from small can.	45%	4	180	260
Sardines, Norway, canned in tomato or mustard sauce, 3-3/4 oz. net from small can.	40%	8	160	240
Sauerkraut, canned, 1/2 cup.	2%	20	2	20
Sauerkraut juice, canned, 6 oz., 3/4 cup.	2%	15	–	15

*See note, p. 46.

	Protein* (% of U.S. RDA)	Carbohydrate Calories	Fat Calories	Total Calories
Sausage, blood (blood pudding and blood and tongue sausage), slice, about 1 oz.	8%	–	90	110
Sausage, bockwurst, 1 link, 7 per pound.	15%	2	140	170
Sausage, bologna. (See bologna.)				
Sausage, braunschweiger. (See braunschweiger.)				
Sausage, brown and serve, cooked yield from 1 patty (1 oz.).	8%	2	80	100
Sausage, brown and serve, cooked yield from 1 link (3/4 oz.).	6%	2	60	70
Sausage, capicola, 3/4 oz. slice from package.	10%	–	90	110
Sausage, cervelat, dry, about 9-1/2 slices, thin, from roll 1-1/2" diam., 1 oz.	15%	2	100	130
Sausage, country style, from 4 oz. raw.	20%	–	320	390
Sausage, frankfurters, without binders, from various meats, about 5" × 7/8", 2 oz.	15%	6	130	170
Sausage, frankfurters, without binders, from various meats, 5" × 3/4", about 1.6 oz. each.	15%	4	100	130

*See note, p. 46.

	Protein* (% of U.S. RDA)	Carbohydrate Calories	Fat Calories	Total Calories
Sausage, frankfurter, without binders, from various meats, cocktail size, about 1/3 oz.	2%	2	25	30
Sausage, frankfurter, with nonfat dried milk or cereal, 5" × 3/4", 1.6 oz.	15%	6	100	140
Sausage, knockwurst, 2.4 oz.	20%	6	140	190
Sausage, liverwurst, 1 oz. slice.	10%	2	70	90
Sausage, mortadella, 1 slice, about 1 oz.	15%	—	60	90
Sausage, Polish, 5-3/8" long, 1" diam., about 2.7 oz.	25%	4	180	230
Sausage, pork, cooked, from 1 oz. link.	6%	—	50	60
Sausage, pork, cooked, about 4" diam. × 1/4" (2 oz.) raw.	10%	—	110	130
Sausage, pork, canned, 2 links, 1 oz.	10%	2	70	90
Sausage, pork, smoked links. (See sausage, country style.)				
Sausage, salami, dry, 6 slices, 1-3/4" diam., × 1/8" thick, 1 oz.	15%	2	100	130
Sausage, salami, cooked, 1 slice from roll 4-1/2" diam., 1 oz.	10%	2	70	90

*See note, p. 46.

	Protein* (% of U.S. RDA)	Carbohydrate Calories	Fat Calories	Total Calories
Sausage, Thuringer, Cervelat or summer sausage, slice from roll 4-3/8″ diam., × 1/8″ thick, 1 oz.	10%	2	60	80
Sausage, Vienna, canned, 2 sausages, about 1 oz.	10%	–	60	80
Scallops, bay and sea, cooked, 1/4 lb.	60%	–	15	120
Scallops, sea scallops, frozen, breaded, fried, reheated, 11 average scallops from random pack, about 4 oz.	45%	50	80	210
Scrapple. (See luncheon meat.)				
Sesame oil. (See oils.)				
Sesame seeds, 1 tbsp.	2%	6	40	50
Shad, baked, 4 oz. cooked (yield from 1/3 lb. raw whole).	60%	–	120	230
Shallot, raw, chopped, 1 tbsp.	–	6	–	8
Sherbet, orange, 3/4 cup, 6 oz.	2%	180	15	200
Shrimp, French fried, 3 oz.	40%	35	80	190
Shrimp, canned, 25 shrimp, 3 oz.	45%	2	10	90
Shrimp, canned, baby, 3-1/2 oz.	30%	2	6	70
Shrimp cocktail, canned, 3-1/2 oz.	10%	70	4	90

*See note, p. 46.

	Protein* (% of U.S. RDA)	Carbohydrate Calories	Fat Calories	Total Calories
Shrimp cakes, frozen, 1 cake, 2 oz.	20%	70	55	160
Shrimp or lobster paste, canned, 1 tsp.	4%	–	6	15
Syrup, maple, 1 tbsp.	–	50	–	50
Syrup, sorghum, 1 tbsp.	–	60	–	60
Syrup, table blends, mainly corn syrup, light or dark, 1 tbsp.	–	60	–	60
Syrup, cane and maple blends (most common of widely sold "maple" syrups).	–	50	–	50

SOUPS: *All 1 cup portions; all prepared with equal volume of water unless specified otherwise.*

Soup, asparagus, cream of, canned.	4%	40	15	60
Soup, asparagus, cream of, canned, prepared with milk.	15%	70	50	150
Soup, bean with pork, canned.	15%	90	50	170
Soup, beef broth, bouillon or consomme, canned.	10%	10	–	30
Soup, beef noodle, canned.	6%	30	25	70
Soup, cream of celery, canned.	2%	35	45	90
Soup, cream of celery, canned, prepared with milk.	15%	60	80	170

*See note, p. 46.

	Protein* (% of U.S. RDA)	Carbohydrate Calories	Fat Calories	Total Calories
Soup, chicken consomme, canned.	6%	8	–	20
Soup, cream of chicken, canned.	6%	30	50	90
Soup, cream of chicken, canned, prepared with milk.	15%	60	90	180
Soup, chicken gumbo, canned.	10%	60	30	110
Soup, chicken noodle, canned.	15%	60	35	130
Soup, chicken with rice, canned.	10%	45	25	90
Soup, chicken vegetable, canned.	15%	80	45	160
Soup, clam chowder, manhattan type, tomatoes, no milk, canned.	8%	100	50	170
Soup, minestrone, canned.	15%	120	60	220
Soup, cream of mushroom, canned.	4%	40	90	130
Soup, cream of mushroom, canned, prepared with milk.	15%	60	130	220
Soup, onion, canned.	8%	20	20	70
Soup, green pea, canned.	8%	90	20	130
Soup, green pea, canned, prepared with milk.	20%	120	60	210
Soup, tomato, canned.	–	15	6	20
Soup, tomato, canned, prepared with milk.	15%	90	60	170
Soup, turkey noodle, canned.	8%	35	25	80

*See note, p. 46.

	Protein* (% of U.S. RDA)	Carbohydrate Calories	Fat Calories	Total Calories
Soup, vegetable beef, canned.	10%	40	20	90
Soup, vegetable with beef broth, canned.	4%	50	15	80
Soup, vegetarian vegetable, canned.	4%	50	20	80
Soup, dehydrated, beef noodle, prepared, 2 oz. pkg. in 3 cups water.	4%	45	10	70
Soup, dehydrated, chicken noodle, prepared, 2 oz. pkg. in 4 cups water.	4%	30	15	50
Soup, dehydrated, chicken rice, prepared, 1-1/2 oz. pkg. in 3 cups water.	2%	35	10	50
Soup, dehydrated, onion, prepared, 1-1/2 oz. pkg. in 4 cups water.	2%	20	10	35
Soup, dehydrated, green pea, prepared, 3 oz. pkg. in 3 cups water.	10%	80	15	120
Soup, dehydrated, tomato vegetable with noodles, prepared 2-1/2 oz. pkg. in 4 cups water.	2%	50	15	70
Soybeans, mature, cooked, 2/3 cup.	20%	80	90	230
Soybean sprouts, raw or cooked, 1/2 cup.	6%	10	6	25
Soybean curd (Tofu), piece 2-1/4" square × 1" thick, 4.2 oz.	15%	10	45	90
Soybean flour, full fat, 1 cup, not stirred.	50%	100	160	360

*See note, p. 46.

	Protein* (% of U.S. RDA)	Carbohydrate Calories	Fat Calories	Total Calories
Soybean flour, low fat, 1 cup.	60%	140	50	310
Soybean flour, defatted, 1 cup.	70%	150	8	330
Soy oils. (See oils.)				
Soy sauce, 1 tbsp.	2%	6	2	10
Soy sauce, 1/2 cup.	10%	60	15	100
Spaghetti, enriched or unenriched, (regular, thin, vermicelli), cooked to firm stage *(al dente),* 1 cup, yield from about 1.8 oz. of dry noodles.	10%	160	6	190
Spaghetti in tomato sauce with cheese, from home recipe, 1 cup.	15%	150	80	260
Spaghetti in tomato sauce with cheese, canned, 1 cup	10%	150	15	190
Spaghetti with meatballs and tomato sauce, home recipe, portion (a little more than two cups, about 1-1/3 cups spaghetti, cooked *al dente,* with about 2/3 cup meatballs and sauce, topped with 2 tbsp. Parmesan cheese).	70%	340	220	720
Spaghetti with meat balls and tomato sauce, canned, regular noodles or rings, portion (one no. 300 can, about 1-3/4 cups, with 4 to 6 meatballs).	40%	190	160	440

*See note, p. 46.

	Protein * (% of U.S. RDA)	Carbohydrate Calories	Fat Calories	Total Calories	
Spaghetti, canned with sausage (franks) 3-1/2 oz.	8%	45	60	130	
Spanish rice, from home recipe, 2/3 cup.	4%	110	40	210	
Spinach, raw, cut up, 1 cup.	2%	10	2	15	
Spinach, fresh, cooked, 2/3 cup.	6%	15	4	25	
Spinach, canned, 2/3 cup.	6%	20	8	35	
Spinach, frozen, chopped or leaf, cooked, 2/3 cup.	6%	20	4	30	
Spinach, creamed, frozen, 3-1/2 oz.	4%	25	40	70	
Spinach, frozen in butter sauce, 3-1/2 oz.	4%	10	25	45	
Spinach, New Zealand, cooked, 1 cup.	4%	15	4	25	
Spot, baked, 4 oz.	60%	–	220	340	
Squash, yellow, crookneck or straightneck, raw or cooked, cut up 2/3 cup.	2%	15	2	20	
Squash, scallop varieties, white or pale green, raw or cooked, cut up, 2/3 cup.	2%	20	–	20	
Squash, zucchini and cocozelle, raw or cooked, cut up, 2/3 cup.	2%	15	–	15	
Squash, acorn, 1/2 squash, baked, a little less than 1 cup.	4%	110	2	110	
Squash, acorn, boiled, 1 cup.	4%	80	2	80	
Squash, butternut, baked, mashed, 1 cup.	6%	140	2	140	

*See note, p. 46.

	Protein* (% of U.S. RDA)	Carbohydrate Calories	Fat Calories	Total Calories
Squash, butternut, boiled, mashed, 1 cup.	4%	100	2	100
Squash, hubbard, baked, mashed, 1 cup.	6%	100	8	110
Squash, hubbard, boiled, mashed, 1 cup.	4%	70	6	80
Squash, winter, frozen, cooked, 1 cup.	4%	90	6	90
Squash, zucchini, frozen, 3-1/2 oz.	2%	10	–	20
Squash, zucchini, fried, frozen, 3-1/2 oz.	6%	100	110	220
Squash, zucchini, Parmesan, frozen, 3-1/2 oz.	8%	20	35	80
Strawberries, raw, 2/3 cup.	2%	35	4	35
Strawberries, canned, water pack, no added sugar, 2/3 cup.	2%	35	2	35
Strawberries, frozen added sugar, sliced, 2/3 cup.	2%	190	4	190
Sturgeon, steamed, 4 oz.	60%	–	60	180
Sturgeon, smoked, 2 oz.	40%	–	10	80
Succotash (corn and lima beans) frozen, cooked, 2/3 cup.	8%	90	4	110
Sugar, beet or cane, brown, 1 cup, packed into cup.	–	820	–	820
Sugar, beet or cane, granulated white, 1 cup.	–	770	–	770
Sugar, beet or cane, granulated white, 1 tsp.	–	15	–	15
Sugar, beet or cane, granulated white, 1 tablet or 2 cubes.	–	20	–	20

*See note, p. 46.

	Protein* (% of U.S. RDA)	Carbohydrate Calories	Fat Calories	Total Calories
Sugar, beet or cane, granulated white, 1 restaurant packet.	–	25	–	25
Sugar, beet or cane, powdered, spooned into cup, 1 cup (about 4.3 oz.).	–	460	–	460
Sugar, maple, 1 oz. piece, about 1-1/2" square × 1/2" thick.	–	100	–	100
Sugar-apples (sweetsop), raw pulp, 1 cup.	6%	240	8	240
Sunflower seeds, dry, in hull, 1/4 cup, about 3/4 oz.	4%	10	50	60
Sunflower seeds, dry, hulled seeds, 1/4 cup, about 1.3 oz.	15%	30	150	200
Surinam cherry. (See Pitanga.)				
Sweetbreads (thymus gland), beef, 3 oz.	50%	–	180	270
Sweetbreads (thymus), calf, 3 oz.	60%	–	25	140
Sweetbreads (thymus), lamb, 3 oz.	50%	–	45	150
Sweet potato, all types, baked or boiled in skin, 5" × 2", size before cooking, 1 potato.	4%	160	6	170
Sweet potato, candied, 2 pieces, each about 2-1/2" × 2".	4%	290	60	350
Sweet potato, canned, 2/3 cup pieces.	4%	130	2	140

*See note, p. 46.

	Protein* (% of U.S. RDA)	Carbohydrate Calories	Fat Calories	Total Calories
Sweet potato, dehydrated flakes, prepared with water, 2/3 cup.	2%	150	2	160
Sweet potatoes, candied, frozen, 3-1/2 oz.	2%	190	2	190
Swiss chard. (See chard.)				
Swordfish, broiled with butter, piece 4-1/2" × 2-1/8" × 7/8" about 5 oz.	80%	–	70	240
Tamales, frozen, 2, 6 oz.	15%	100	140	280
Tangelo juice, fresh, 6 oz. glass.	2%	70	2	80
Tangerine, medium, 2-3/8" diam., about 6 oz.	2%	40	2	40
Tangerine juice, fresh or canned, unsweetened, 6 oz. glass.	2%	75	4	80
Tangerine juice, canned, sugar added, 6 oz. glass.	2%	90	6	100
Tangerine juice, from frozen concentrate, prepared, 6 oz. glass.	2%	80	4	90
Tapioca pudding, 2/3 cup.	10%	80	50	150
Tartar sauce, regular, 1 tbsp.	–	2	70	70
Tartar sauce, low calorie, 1 tbsp.	–	4	30	30
Tendergreen. (See mustard spinach.)				
Thuringer. (See sausage.)				
Toaster tarts and pastries, 1 average.	6%	140	50	210
Tomato, green, raw, about 5 oz. or 3 per lb.	2%	30	2	35

*See note, p. 46.

	Protein* (% of U.S. RDA)	Carbohydrate Calories	Fat Calories	Total Calories
Tomato, red ripe, medium, raw, about 5 oz., or 3 per lb.	2%	25	2	30
Tomato, canned, 1 cup.	2%	30	4	50
Tomato catsup, 1 tbsp. or packet, about 1/2 oz.	–	15	–	15
Tomato catsup or chili sauce, 1 tbsp.	–	15	–	15
Tomato juice, 6 oz., canned or bottled.	2%	30	2	35
Tomato juice cocktail, 6 oz. glass.	2%	35	2	40
Tomato paste, canned, 1/2 cup.	8%	95	5	110
Tongue, beef, pork, lamb, cooked, slice about 3″ × 2″ × 1/8″, 3/4 oz.	10%	–	30	50
Tongue, calf, cooked, 3/4 oz. slice, as above.	10%	–	10	30
Tonic water (quinine), sweetened, 12 oz.	–	110	–	110
Tuna, canned in oil, solid pack or chunk style, drained fish from 7 oz. can, 1/2 can, about 3 oz.	50%	–	60	150
Tuna, packed in water, solid pack or chunk style, fish from 7 oz. can, 1/2 can.	60%	–	8	120
Tuna salad (tuna, celery, mayonnaise, pickle, onion and egg), 1/2 cup.	35%	15	100	180

*See note, p. 46.

	Protein* (% of U.S. RDA)	Carbohydrate Calories	Fat Calories	Total Calories
Turkey, roasted, light meat, 2 slices, each 4" × 2" × 1/4", about 3 oz.	60%	–	30	150
Turkey, roasted, dark meat, 4 pieces, each 2-1/2" × 1-5/8" × 1/4", about 3 oz.	60%	–	60	170
Turkey, canned (or in a jar), half of 5-1/2 oz. can, solid pack, 2-3/4 oz.	35%	–	90	160
Turkey giblets, cooked, 1/2 cup.	35%	4	100	170
Turkey dinner, frozen, 11–12 oz.	50%	190	50	380
Turkey in giblet gravy, frozen entree, 1/2 of boil-in-bag, about 2-1/2 oz.	70%	45	20	230
Turkey, potted. (See luncheon meat.)				
Turkey potpie, home recipe, about 8 oz.	50%	170	280	540
Turkey roast, rolled, frozen, 3-1/2 oz.	70%	2	90	220
Turnips, fresh, cooked, 2/3 cup, cut up.	2%	20	2	25
Turnip greens, fresh, frozen, canned, cooked, 2/3 cup.	4%	15	2	25
Veal, loin cuts, chuck cuts and boneless veal for stew, cooked, 6 pieces, each 1-1/4" square × 3/4" thick, about 4-1/2 oz.	80%	–	150	300

*See note, p. 46.

	Protein * (% of U.S. RDA)	Carbohydrate Calories	Fat Calories	Total Calories
Veal, rib roast, 3 pieces, each about 4" × 2-1/4" × 1/4", about 4-1/2 oz.	80%	–	190	340
Veal, round and rump, cutlets, cooked, 3 pieces, about 4" × 2" × 1/4", about 4 oz.	80%	–	130	280
Veal cutlet, frozen, Parmigiana style, dinner, about 11-12 oz.	45%	170	170	420
Vegetable juice cocktail, canned, 6 oz. glass.	2%	25	–	30
Vegetables, frozen, Chinese style, 3-1/2 oz.	4%	25	40	70
Vegetables, frozen, Danish style, 3-1/2 oz.	2%	30	70	100
Vegetables, frozen, Florida style, 3-1/2 oz.	2%	20	25	50
Vegetables, frozen, Hawaiian, 3-1/2 oz.	2%	50	50	100
Vegetables, frozen, Italian, 3-1/2 oz.	4%	35	60	100
Vegetables, frozen, Japanese, 3-1/2 oz.	2%	25	80	110
Vegetables, frozen, Mexican, 3-1/2 oz.	8%	70	80	160
Vegetables, frozen, mixed, 3-1/2 oz.	6%	70	4	80
Vegetables, frozen, mixed, butter sauce, 3-1/2 oz.	4%	40	20	70
Vegetables, frozen, New Orleans, 3-1/2 oz.	4%	30	35	70
Vegetables, frozen, Northwest style, 3-1/2 oz.	4%	40	30	80

*See note, p. 46.

	Protein* (% of U.S. RDA)	Carbohydrate Calories	Fat Calories	Total Calories
Vegetables, frozen, Paris style, 3-1/2 oz.	2%	30	60	100
Venison, lean meat only, 6 oz.	80%	–	60	210
Vienna sausage. (See sausage.)				
Waffle, from home recipe or mix, egg and milk added, 4-1/2" square.	8%	80	45	140
Waffle, frozen, 4-5/8" × 3-3/4".	4%	60	20	90
Walnuts, shelled, chopped pieces, 1 tbsp.	2%	4	40	50
Waterchestnut, 2 oz., 2-1/2 to 3 corms.	–	35	4	35
Watercress, 3 sprigs, about 1/3 cup.	–	2	–	2
Watermelon, slice, 1" thick, from melon 10" diam.	4%	110	8	110
Welsh rarebit, 1/2 cup.	20%	30	140	210
Wheat flour, whole, from hard wheat, spooned into 1 cup.	25%	340	20	400
Wheat flour, all purpose, unsifted, 1 cup.	20%	420	15	500
Wheat flour, bread type, unsifted, 1 cup.	25%	410	15	500
Wheat flour, cake or pastry type, unsifted, 1 cup.	15%	370	8	430
Wheat flour. gluten flour, unsifted, 1 cup.	90%	260	25	530
Wheat flour, self-rising type, unsifted, 1 cup.	20%	370	10	440

*See note, p. 46.

	Protein* (% of U.S. RDA)	Carbohydrate Calories	Fat Calories	Total Calories
Wheat cereal, rolled, cooked, 1 cup.	8%	160	10	180
Wheat cereal, whole meal, cooked, 1 cup.	6%	90	6	110
Wheat and malted barley cereal, quickcooking type, 3 min., cooked, 1 cup.	8%	130	6	160
Wheat and malted barley cereal, instant cooking type, cooked, 1 cup.	10%	160	6	200
Wheat bran, ready-to-eat cereal. (See bran.)				
Wheat flakes, ready-to-eat cereal, added sugar, 1 cup, dry.	4%	100	4	110
Wheat germ, toasted, no sugar added, 1 tbsp., dry.	2%	10	6	25
Wheat, puffed ready-to-eat cereal, no sugar, 1 cup dry.	4%	50	2	50
Wheat, puffed ready-to-eat cereal, sugar or sugar and honey added, 1 cup.	4%	120	6	130
Wheat, shredded, ready-to-eat cereal, biscuit about 4" long, no sugar.	4%	80	4	90
Wheat, shredded, spoon-size biscuits, no sugar, 1 cup.	8%	160	10	180
Wheat, shredded bite-size squares with malt and sugar, 1 cup.	8%	180	15	200

*See note, p. 46.

	Protein* (% of U.S. RDA)	Carbohydrate Calories	Fat Calories	Total Calories
Wheat, shredded, shreds with malt and sugar, 1 cup.	6%	130	10	150
Wheat and malted barley flakes, added sugar, 1 cup.	6%	130	4	160
Whitefish, lake, baked, stuffed, 4 oz.	40%	25	140	240
Whitefish, lake, smoked, 4 oz.	50%	–	75	180
White sauce, thin, 1/2 cup.	10%	35	100	150
White sauce, medium, 1/2 cup.	10%	45	140	200
White sauce, thick, 1/2 cup.	10%	60	180	250
Wine. (See beverages, alcoholic.)				
Yam, 8 oz. serving.	6%	180	8	200
Yambean, 8 oz. serving.	4%	100	8	110
Yeast, bakers, compressed, one packet, 1-1/4" square × 3/4" thick, 0.6 oz.	4%	8	–	15
Yeast, dry (active), one packet, about 1/4 oz., scant tbsp.	4%	10	–	20
Yeast, brewer's, debittered, 1 tbsp.	4%	10	–	20
Yeast, torula, 1 oz.	15%	40	2	80
Yogurt, low fat, from partially skimmed milk, 1 cup, 8 oz.	20%	50	40	130
Yogurt, from whole milk, 1 cup.	15%	50	70	150

*See note, p. 46.

	Protein* (% of U.S. RDA)	Carbohydrate Calories	Fat Calories	Total Calories
Yogurt, fruit, 1 cup,	15%	210	40	280
(includes such as apricot, blueberry, cherry, peach, pineapple, strawberry, vanilla, etc.)	15%	210	40	280
Youngberries. (See blackberries.)				
Zwieback, 2 pieces, about 1/2 oz.	2%	40	10	60

*See note, p. 46.

Sample Diet Analysis

As an example, say you are a man who weighs 172 pounds, you work in an office and lead a moderately active life, but you get no particular strenuous exercise, and your doctor has advised you to "lose a few pounds."

You turn to the chart on p. 37, which shows the following for your approximate weight:

Weight	Total Calories
170	2975
180	3150

At 172 pounds, you are closer to 170 than 180, so you would figure you burn up about 3,000 total calories in a day. Furthermore, looking at the chart on p. 39, you see that your fat limit would be about 1050 calories a day (1041 calories for the closest listed calorie total: 2975 calories). And finally, you should aim to get a minimum of about half of your calories (1500 of the 3,000) in carbohydrates.

The next thing is to start keeping track of what you eat — to list the foods, then look them up in the Fat Counter tables and fill in columns for percentage of protein allowance and for calories. Let's say a typical day looks like this:

	Protein (% of U.S. RDA)	Carbohydrate Calories	Fat Calories	Total Calories
BREAKFAST				
Orange juice (1 cup).	2%	115	2	120
Bread (2 slices).	8%	120	16	160
Butter (2 pats).	–	–	80	80
Coffee	–	–	–	–
– 1 tsp. sugar.	–	15	–	15
Corn flakes (1 cup).	4%	90	–	100
– 1 tbsp. sugar.	–	45	–	45
– whole milk (4 oz.).	10%	25	40	80
"DIET LUNCH"				
Hamburger, lean (6 oz.).	100%	–	180	380
Cottage cheese (1/2 cup).	30%	12	40	110
Peaches, canned (1/2 cup).	–	100	4	100
Lettuce.	–	4	–	5
Diet drink.	–	–	–	–
SNACK				
Brownies, 2.	4%	80	120	200
Milk, whole (8 oz.).	20%	50	80	160
DINNER				
Beef, rib roast (6 oz. untrimmed).	80%	–	600	750
Potato, baked.	6%	130	2	140
– butter (2 pats).	–	–	80	80
Salad, lettuce.	–	4	–	5
– dressing (2 tbsp.)	–	8	160	160
Biscuit.	3%	50	45	100
– butter (1 pat).	–	–	40	40
Pie, apple.	4%	180	120	300
TOTAL	271%	1028	1609	3130

You can see that (1) you are getting far more protein than you need, (2) you are getting considerably more of your calories in fat and considerably less in carbohydrates than is probably best for you, and (3) you are apparently getting a few more total calories than your body is burning up (and will be gradually gaining weight instead of losing as you'd hoped).

A quick check shows items on your menu that are contributing substantial fat and a lot of calories. Surprisingly, they include some of the "high protein" foods so often associated with popular reducing diets. The typical "diet lunch" doesn't look very useful in terms of fats and total calories. Other candidates for change are the untrimmed beef, the whole milk, the salad dressing, and the butter on the potatoes.

Say you made some changes in those foods, concentrating on alternatives which are lower in fat but just as appetizing. You could trim the fat from the beef, switch to skim milk, and substitute a bacon-lettuce-and-tomato sandwich and a glass of skim milk for the "diet lunch." You could pick another green vegetable, say snap beans, which does not carry the fat calorie burden of the salad dressing. You could also replace the butter on the potato with zesty yogurt. This would change the picture as follows:

	Protein (% of U.S. RDA)	Carbohydrate Calories	Fat Calories	Total Calories
Instead of:				
Untrimmed beef (6 oz.).	80%	–	600	750
Whole milk (with snack).	20%	50	80	160
Butter (on potatoes).	–	–	80	80
Salad, lettuce.	–	4	–	5
– dressing.	–	8	160	160
"DIET LUNCH"				
– hamburger.	100%	–	180	380
– cottage cheese.	30%	12	40	110
– peaches.	–	100	4	100
– lettuce.	–	4	–	5
TOTAL SUBTRACTED	230%	178	1144	1750
You Will Get:				
Trimmed beef (4 oz.).	70%	–	140	280
Skim milk (with snack).	20%	50	2	90
Yogurt (2 tbsp.)	2%	2	5	15
Snap beans (2/3 cup).	2%	20	–	25
NEW LUNCH				
– bacon (2 slices).	8%	2	70	90
– bread (2 slices).	8%	120	16	160
– mayonnaise (1/2 tbsp.)	–	–	50	50
– tomato (1/2).	–	12	–	15
– lettuce.	–	4	–	5
– skim milk (8 oz.).	20%	50	2	90
TOTAL ADDED	130%	260	285	820
Which Means a Net Change of	–100%	+82	–859	–930

	Protein (% of U.S. RDA)	Carbohydrate Calories	Fat Calories	Total Calories
Adding to (or subtracting from) the original diet totals, you find that you now get:				
Original Diary Totals	271%	1028	1609	3130
Net Change	−100%	+82	−859	−930
New Totals	171%	1110	750	2200
Percent of Total Calories		(50%)	(34%)	

What have you accomplished? You have eliminated a diet high in fat and low in carbohydrates, which contributed far more protein than you could use, and on which you would probably gain weight. You have created a new diet, which meets the fat-carbohydrate goals, still provides ample protein, and on which you will eventually lose a lot of weight (about 1-1/2 pounds per week).

Total calories have dropped to a level where you now show a daily deficit of about 800 calories. You have actually beaten your weight-reduction goal. And now, even if you can't resist that donut at the coffee break, you'll still lose a pound a week. You've made room for a treat.

Of course, your diet will vary, and you probably won't want to add up every item every day. But periodic samplings will show you how you are doing and the Fat Counter will show you the alternatives which will help you achieve your objectives. You've learned a way to make choices. And choice is what practical nutrition is all about.

OTHER POPULAR BOOKS ON NUTRITION AND HEALTH

- [ ] **Realities of Nutrition** (cloth) 405 pp.
  by Ronald M. Deutsch   @$10.95

- [ ] **Realities of Nutrition** (paper) 405 pp.
  by Ronald M. Deutsch   @$ 7.50

- [ ] **New Nuts Among the Berries** (paper) 350 pp.
  by Ronald M. Deutsch,   @$ 4.95

- [ ] **Food for Sport** (paper) 188 pp.
  by Nathan J. Smith, M.D.   @$ 4.95

- [ ] **Habits, Not Diets** (paper) 252 pp.
  by James M. Ferguson, M.D.   @$ 7.95

- [ ] **I Almost Feel Thin** (paper) 182 pp.
  by Albert J. Stunkard, M.D.   @$ 5.95

- [ ] **Just One More** (paper) 193 pp.
  by James L. Free   @$ 4.95

- [ ] **The Fat Counter Diet** (paper) 160 pp.
  by Ronald M. Deutsch   @$ 3.95
  Please send and bill me for a copy upon publication.

Bull Publishing Co., P.O. Box 208, Palo Alto CA 94302

Please send me the books I have checked above.

- [ ] Bill me, adding freight and 50¢ handling charge.
- [ ] Check enclosed. (Save freight and handling.)
  (Calif. residents add 6% sales tax.)

Name _____

Street _____

City _____ State _____ Zip _____